Seating and Mobility

For Persons with
Physical Disabilities

. . . .

by

Elaine Trefler, M.Ed., OTR, FAOTA
Douglas A. Hobson, Ph.D.
Susan Johnson Taylor, B.S., OTR/L
Lynn C. Monahan, M.P.A., OTR
C. Greg Shaw, M.Sc.

for the University of Tennessee Rehabilitation
Engineering Program

Text Illustrations drawn under contract by
Corwyn Zimbleman

Therapy Skill Builders
A division of
Communication Skill Builders ®
3830 E. Bellevue/P.O. Box 42050
Tucson, Arizona 85733/(602) 323-7500

Reproducing Pages from This Book

Some pages in this book can be reproduced for administrative use (not for resale). To protect your book, make a photocopy of each reproducible page. Then use that copy as a master for photocopying or other types of reproduction.

Published by

Therapy Skill Builders
A division of
Communication Skill Builders ®
3830 E. Bellevue/P.O. Box 42050
Tucson, Arizona 85733/(602) 323-7500

ISBN 0-88450-598-7   Catalog No. 4726

10 9 8 7 6 5 4 3
Printed in the United States of America

For information about our audio and/or video products, write us at:
Therapy Skill Builders, P.O. Box 42050, Tucson, AZ 85733.

Acknowledgments

The authors would like to thank the clients and their families who taught us so much about people and technology.

Dr. Robert Tooms and Ms. Margaret Hyde provided us with guidance and the freedom to be creative.

Beverly, Linda, Hope, and Peggy kept us accountable.

And thanks as well to our many colleagues who kept asking questions which forced us to look for answers.

About the Authors

Elaine Trefler, M.Ed., OTR, FAOTA, is a private consultant in assistive technology in Pittsburgh, Pennsylvania, and an assistant professor in the department of Rehabilitation Science and Technology, University of Pittsburgh. She has worked for more than 20 years in the field of rehabilitation engineering at the Hugh MacMillan Medical Centre in Toronto, the Rehabilitation Centre for Children in Winnipeg, and the University of Tennessee Rehabilitation Engineering Program in Memphis. Her areas of special interest are the application of assistive technology for both adults and children, including seating and mobility systems, augmentative communication devices, and computer access.

Ms. Trefler graduated from the University of Toronto in physical and occupational therapy. She received a B.O.T. from the University of Manitoba in Winnipeg, and an M.Ed. from Memphis State University. In 1988 she was made a Fellow of the American Occupational Therapy Association for her contribution in the area of assistive technology.

Douglas A. Hobson, Ph.D., is currently associate professor and Director, Rehabilitation Technology Program in the Department of Rehabilitation Science and Technology, School of Health and Rehabilitation Sciences, University of Pittsburgh. From 1990 to 1992, he was the President and CEO of the Canadian Aging and Rehabilitation Product Development Corporation in Winnipeg, Canada. He began the Rehabilitation Engineering Program, University of Tennessee in 1974 within the Department of Orthopedic Surgery. It was a program in which many of the seating principles and systems were developed and shared by others in the field.

Dr. Hobson received his undergraduate degree in mechanical engineering from the University of Manitoba and his Ph.D. in bioengineering from the University of Strathclyde in Glasgow, Scotland. His dissertation research was on the relationship between sitting posture and the seat interface pressure and shear factors.

Susan Johnson Taylor, B.S., OTR/L, has worked in the field of rehabilitation technology for more than 12 years. Receiving a B.S. in occupational therapy from Boston University, she has worked with the University of Tennessee Rehabilitation Engineering Program and with a supplier of rehabilitation technology. Currently she is occupational therapy pediatric coordinator of seating clinic staff at Shepherd Spinal Center in Atlanta.

Ms. Taylor is actively involved with RESNA, including the Education Committee and the Meetings Committee, of which she is the Instructional Program Chair. She also serves on the professional advisory committee of Team Rehab.

Lynn C. Monahan, M.P.A., OTR, is currently the director of the Seating/Mobility Service of United Medical in Memphis, Tennessee. When she was an occupational therapist with the University of Tennessee Rehabilitation Engineering Program, she was involved in assessing and providing seating systems, mobility aids, and technical devices for individuals with severe disabilities.

Ms. Monahan received a B.S. in occupational therapy from Eastern Kentucky University, and an M.P.A. in public administration from Memphis State University.

C. Greg Shaw, M.Sc., is a rehabilitation engineer who has served as both the director of client services and acting technical director for the University of Tennessee Rehabilitation Engineering Program. He has also served as the vice president of the Center for Design/Project Enable, a pilot effort to help people with disabilities via volunteer help. He is currently a research scientist at the University of Virginia Rehabilitation Engineering Center, and a senior rehabilitation engineer for product research and development.

Mr. Shaw received a B.S. and an M.Sc. in mechanical engineering from Stanford University. He is presently working on a Ph.D. in bioengineering from Strathclyde University in Glasgow, Scotland.

Contents

Introduction

This manual was written as a guide for clinicians and technical personnel challenged by the seating and positioning needs of persons with physical disabilities.

Rationale

For many years, the staff of the Rehabilitation Engineering Program at the University of Tennessee—Memphis have been involved in training workshops for professionals from all over the world, and much of the material in this book has evolved from the lectures and handouts prepared for those courses.

With each workshop and seminar, it became evident that there are always professionals who need training in the basics—that the technology is available, but the question is how to evaluate clients and help them to decide what is the most appropriate technology for them.

The content of this manual is geared to help clinicians develop the skills to be good evaluators and problem solvers for their clients who require seating and mobility technology.

Organization of This Manual

This book is divided into several sections. The first part, General Concerns of Seating and Mobility, includes chapters on the development of wheelchair technology, basic biomechanical principles as they relate to the seating field, and mobility considerations for persons with disabilities.

The second section of the book, Evaluation and Prescription Principles and Practices, includes chapters on evaluation and the special seating and mobility considerations of persons with specific disabilities (cerebral palsy, head injury, muscular dystrophy, and spinal cord injury [both acquired and congenital]), and the special needs of elderly persons who use wheelchairs.

The appendixes include a standardized terminology listing and information about the types and specific manufacturers of the technology described in the book.

Scope of the Text

Seating and Mobility for Persons with Physical Disabilities reflects the collective experiences and opinions of the authors. For this reason, there is no information on the needs of persons with multiple sclerosis or on those who have suffered a stroke. These people were not often referred to the clinic at UTREP and therefore we have no special expertise related to their needs. However, the process of problem solving and decision making for these people would follow the same lines as for others, and much information can be gleaned from reading other chapters.

It is the intent of the authors to provide a guide to problem solving, not the solutions. With the process of evaluation and decision making in place and the technology choices available either in the commercial sector or the seating workshops, we believe that cost-effective, functional seating and mobility systems are possible for all who need them.

Development of Wheelchair Technology*

*Reprinted with permission from: Hobson, D. A. 1988. Seating and mobility for the severely disabled. In *Rehabilitation engineering,* edited by J. Leslie, 193-200, 237-239. Copyright, CRC Press, Inc., Boca Raton, Florida.

Development of Wheelchair Technology

It has been estimated that, in the United States, approximately 750,000 people with disabilities use some form of personal wheeled mobility, such as a traditional wheelchair. Most are unable to walk; some have difficulty walking and therefore may use the device for only short periods of time. The majority have chronic disabilities that require the daily use of a mobility device for the remainder of their lives. Of the 750,000, it is further estimated that 10% to 15% use electrically (battery) powered devices (Wilson 1986).

Historical Overview

Early Developments

The early history of wheelchairs remains somewhat obscure. Patent records indicate that designs similar to the present configurations of user-propelled wheelchairs date back to 1894 (Wilson 1986). In 1932, Herbert A. Everest, a mining engineer with a disability, and Harry C. Jennings, a mechanical engineer, teamed up to design and patent the present-day cross (X) frame folding wheelchair (figure 1). They went on to form Everest and Jennings Inc., which is one of the largest international manufacturers of wheelchairs today. Their patent was registered in the United States patent office in October, 1937 (Everest and Jennings 1937).

The development of the X-frame folding wheelchair rapidly replaced the pre-existing wooden-seat, nonfolding design, especially for nonambulatory people wanting a lightweight wheelchair that would fold small enough to be transported in an automobile. Probably no other single development has influenced personal wheeled mobility as much as the Everest and Jennings design—it became the standard for the industry that exists to this day.

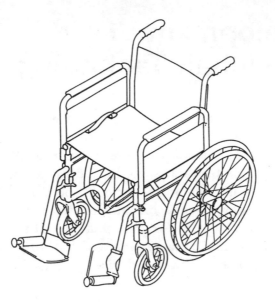

Figure 1. Traditional cross frame (X-frame) folding wheel-chair with sling upholstery seat and back. *(Courtesy of Rehabilitation Press)*

Over the decades, the folding X-frame design has met the needs of a large number of people with disabilities. Those requiring temporary use of a wheelchair, or those having relatively normal upper-body function who can manually propel the large drive wheels (such as people with paraplegia) have derived tremendous benefits from the flexibility of the traditional folding wheelchair.

However, other populations of people with disabilities have needs for more intimate upper-body support, body posturing, externally powered mobility, recreation mobility, transportation while in the wheelchair, or pressure relief over weight-bearing areas. To a significant extent, the needs of these latter populations were compromised by the industry dominance of the basic folding X-frame design.

To minimize the weight of the wheelchair and achieve ease of folding, the Everest and Jennings design utilized vinyl sling-type upholstery to replace the firm seat and back components used by its predecessors. Sling-type support surfaces do not provide the degree of support or stability needed by individuals lacking trunk stability and upper extremity function. Since there is no adjustability to sling-type support surfaces, alteration of body posture to positions different from those imposed by the sling surfaces is difficult.

The sling seat does not distribute pressures well for those who must be concerned about the onset of pressure sores due to insensitive tissue underlying the weight-bearing areas of the pelvis. Additionally, this type of seat fails to provide a platform for equal weight distribution for persons who have asymmetrical tone or accommodation for those with orthopedic involvement. For those lacking the upper-body function necessary to propel the wheelchairs, the large rear drive wheels serve little useful function other than to negotiate obstacles such as curbs when propelled by an attendant.

Powered Wheelchairs
. . . .

Electrically powered wheelchairs are a more recent development. Although an early design was patented in 1940 (Smith 1940), common use did not occur until 1957. In an effort to broaden the use of wheelchairs, motors, controls, and car batteries were added to the Everest and Jennings folding frame (figure 2). This development rapidly became the industry standard for powered mobility which largely remains to this day.

Although the addition of the powered components renders the wheelchair heavy and non-foldable for all practical purposes, the X-frame design and the sling-type support surfaces were retained. Powered mobility has given large numbers of people with disabilities increased independence in their mobility and lifestyle. However, posturing needs became even more acute since most people who require powered mobility also have need for increased upper-body support.

Mechanics of Manually Powered Mobility

Over the past decade, a number of studies have investigated the factors affecting the performance of rim-propelled wheelchairs. Studies on the effects of rolling resistance (Brubaker 1986), propulsion efficiency, location of center of gravity and

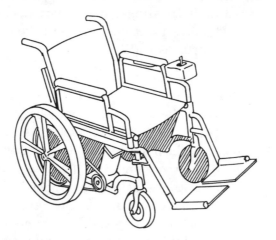

Figure 2. Traditional battery-powered (X-frame) electric wheelchair. *(Courtesy of Rehabilitation Press)*

body position relative to drive wheels (Brubaker, McClay, and McLaurin 1984a), and the effects of mechanical advantage on propulsion efficiency (Brubaker, McClay, and McLaurin 1984b) emphasize the advantages of the new generation of ultralight wheelchairs over the traditional wheelchair in terms of improved interface between person and machine and overall biomechanical performance.

Other studies have evaluated the use of lever drives as an alternative method of propelling a wheelchair. One study presented results on EMG (electromyographic) analysis of lever placement (Brubaker, McLaurin, and McClay 1985), and another study discussed the mechanics of a lever-drive prototype design (McLaurin and Brubaker 1986). A three-dimensional model of a lever propulsion system has also been developed and reported upon (Sheth and Brubaker 1987).

Several other studies have analyzed the dynamic performance of a wheelchair, including the factors affecting rolling resistance, caster shimmy, and the control stability of wheelchairs with rear-mounted casters (Collins and Kauzlarich 1987; Kauzlarich, Bruning, and Thacker, 1983; Kauzlarich and Thacker 1985). Others have investigated the effects of side slopes on wheelchair performance (Brubaker, McLaurin, and McClay 1986) and the effects of the speed regulation in rim propulsion (Woude, Veeger, and Rozendal 1987).

Finally, it is exciting to see an increasing number of hand-propelled recreation tricycles becoming commercially available. A recent study has compared four developments in which performance features such as braking distance, turning radius, stability, and speed were compared (Segner and Bergstrand 1987). The Veterans Administration has published an excellent supplement to their *Journal of Rehabilitation Research and Development* which features physical fitness and increased opportunities for those interested in recreational and sports mobility devices (Kegel 1985).

Electromechanical Developments in Powered Mobility

Since November 1956, when the first belt-drive, microswitch-controlled, 12-volt model of powered wheelchairs became available (Everest and Jennings model #834), significant developments have taken place. These developments have occurred within seven distinct areas: an expanded user demand, evaluation tools, improved control options, integrated controls, alternative drive trains, investigation of new energy sources, and the advent of microprocessor control systems.

Recently there has been a growing trend towards powered mobility for younger and younger children, especially those with severe physical disabilities. Traditional therapeutic practices suggest that if children could ambulate at all or propel a manual wheelchair at all, they should be encouraged to do so. This depressed the market for child-sized powered devices and, therefore, very few commercial options for children existed even as recently as 1980. But recent studies have shown the importance of providing young children with the means for functional independent mobility (Taylor 1986; Trefler and Marcrum 1987). Independent mobility is particularly important in improving general attitudes and body image, as well as improving social skills through increased peer activities.

The quest for increased independence—which includes mobility—by adults with severe disabilities has created a demand for improved control options, that is, options for controlling the wheelchair that go beyond traditional joystick control. Chin and head controls, optical head pointers, touch switches, single switch scanning control, sip and puff, and voice-activated controls are among the new options that can now be used by people who have little or no use of the upper limbs.

Provision of powered mobility for individuals with very limited upper-body function creates a special decision-making challenge for the provision team. Since powered mobility devices with advanced control options are usually expensive, it is important to be able to evaluate a user's potential ability to control a particular device prior to making a financial commitment.

This evaluation need has spawned a parallel development area concerned with the evaluation of motor, perceptual, and cognitive factors influencing mobility control. Research efforts in this area have identified batteries of standardized tests (Verburg, Field, and Jarvis 1987) and developed computer-based simulation tests and actual driving simulators (Taylor 1986) that are beginning to quantify a person's potential to safely control a powered wheelchair.

Many people with severe disabilities have the need to control multiple devices including a powered wheelchair, electronic communication aids, a computer keyboard, and possibly an environmental control device. The new generation wheelchair controllers (in particular, the models that are microprocessor-based) provide the opportunity of controlling all these activities from the powered wheelchair (Brown and Inigo 1987; Shire 1987; Trefler, Nickey, and Hobson 1987). These advanced options can be termed "integrated control options" which are now becoming available in several commercial models of wheelchairs.

Several projects have studied the electromechanical characteristics of the wheelchair control system. Electromechanical braking, velocity feedback, acceleration damping (bucking prevention), electronic spasticity damping, and improved energy conversion efficiency are but a few of the recent innovations being studied for wheelchair control systems (Antczak and Snell 1987; Inigo and Kim 1987; Jagacinski et al. 1987; Smith et al. 1984).

Similar studies have been carried out to improve the reliability and safety of microprocessor-based controllers. Sensitivity to power fluctuations and safe recovery from transit disturbances in order to permit safe operation under stringent user conditions have also been studied (Johnson, Aylor, and Williams 1987).

The liquid electrolyte, deep cycle, lead-acid battery has been the primary power source for powered mobility devices from the very beginning. Alternate lead-acid batteries (Kauzlarich and Junkmann 1987) as well as different gel electrolyte batteries (Fisher, Garrett, and Seeger 1988) have been compared for use in wheelchairs. Also, improved methods of monitoring battery condition for purposes of recharging and/or making replacement decisions have been sought (Aylor and Lim 1987).

Most electrically powered wheelchairs use some form of direct drive involving belts, chains, and/or gears. On a smooth, level surface, relatively little torque is required to propel the wheelchair and occupant at constant speeds up to five or six miles per hour. In actual use, wheelchairs must overcome obstacles at low speeds, climb substantial grades, turn on soft terrains, and accelerate at a reasonable rate.

Most of these conditions demand high torque at low speeds. In order to obtain both the high and low speeds performance with a fixed speed ratio drive train, large motors and energy sources are required. As a result, the motors are operating at reduced efficiency much of the time because high torque is obtained only at low speed.

Reswick (1985) has reported the development of an automatic transmission that has infinitely variable power transmission capability, which automatically changes its speed ratio in response to the torque being transmitted. The substantial reduction in operating current and overall energy consumption yields improved efficiencies and increased range of operation, when compared to the traditional direct-drive chair using the same battery charge.

In summary, significant electromechanical advances are taking place in powered mobility options, especially for the young and those with severe disabilities. However, much remains to be done. The next decade should see many of these prototype developments being made available in a wide range of new commercial powered mobility products.

Safety Issues

The conventional X-frame wheelchair was never designed to be used as a device to transport people in vans or school buses. The advent of school busing laws and the quest for more independent life styles by people with severe disabilities has meant that conventional wheelchairs are now being used in vans and buses. The problem remains unresolved from the safety perspective, since it has been demonstrated in simulated crash tests that most conventional wheelchair designs and their often make-shift restraint devices will not withstand the destructive forces generated under crash conditions (Seeger and Luxton 1984).

Ultralights

In the late 1970s, a design revolution began in the wheelchair industry—the ultralight wheelchair. The impetus for change came largely from the needs of people with disabilities who engaged in wheelchair athletics. They needed higher-performance and lighter-weight equipment to be more competitive. This need spawned a series of design alternatives which are now being used in new designs for both children and adults not necessarily engaged in athletic activity.

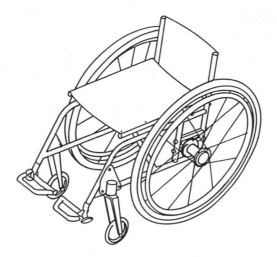

Figure 3. A contemporary ultralight wheelchair. *(Courtesy of Rehabilitation Press)*

Many of these designs have moved away from the X-frame folding concept towards fixed frames, adjustable wheel bases, and firmer body support surfaces (figure 3). In general, the back supports have been lowered, which works well for people with good upper body function. However, this still leaves an unmet need for those who require more intimate body support, significant pressure relief, and posturing of the body in positions other than those imposed by the commercial ultralight wheelchairs.

The quest for higher performance in manually propelled mobility also encouraged researchers to study the biomechanics of wheelchair propulsion and the mechanical factors of rolling resistance, wheeled base configurations, and newer structural materials that could lead to improved efficiencies of motion. More recent studies have been done on battery performance, power train design, base configuration, and efficiency of electronic control devices in an effort to improve the functional performance of powered wheelchairs.

Pressure Relief

Relief of pressure acting on insensitive tissue or relief of discomfort resulting from prolonged sitting is vitally important to segments of the nonambulatory population. Injuries to the spinal cord can render people partially or totally paralyzed in their lower limbs, as well as asensitive below the level of the spinal lesion. Interface pressures, especially if sustained over prolonged periods of time, can occlude (restrict) the blood supply to supporting tissues.

Excessive pressures, combined with other factors such as excessive heat and humidity buildup, nutritional and systematic deficiencies, and possibly repeated impact loadings to the more susceptible areas, can lead to tissue breakdown and onset of pressure sores. If severe, pressure sores can require surgical intervention or possibly even lead to death if deep tissue infection is also present.

A wheelchair cushion industry has developed in an attempt to resolve these pressure-related problems. A variety of technological approaches have been undertaken to remove or reduce the pressures in the more susceptible areas of the supporting pelvic surface tissues and underlying bony structures. These commercial developments have largely taken the form of cushions that are placed on the sling seat surfaces of conventional wheelchairs. They are also used with the newer ultralight designs.

The primary purpose of these cushions has been the reduction of seat interface pressures. For many within this need group, these cushions have worked well. However, it is only recently that the cushion industry has given attention to the needs for upper body support or posturing.

Other groups of people, such as those with muscular dystrophy, those who have had polio, and elderly people, often lack the ability to alter their body posture to obtain relief from discomfort resulting from prolonged sitting in one posture. The cushions developed for pressure relief have been used fairly successfully by those seeking relief from discomfort in the buttock tissues. Again, these developments had not traditionally addressed the problems of upper body support or body posturing in these populations.

Upper Body and Posture Support
· ·

In the mid-1960s, clinicians and designers were stimulated by the needs of still another large population of people with physical disabilities, mainly children with cerebral palsy, spina bifida, and other less common congenital disorders. Many within this population, especially those with cerebral palsy, required total body posturing, a feature that was not available in commercially available devices at that time.

The sling-type seat and back support surfaces often do not provide the posturing support needed. Traditional wheelchair designs do not allow independent adjustments to positions of the body segments relevant to each other or alignment of the whole body in space. For many individuals, alternate wheeled bases were necessary, since self-propulsion was not possible and total body tilt features were necessary.

Accessories to support head, feet, and arms were also necessary. Many individuals had tonal problems or involuntary muscle activity that made retention in the desirable posture very difficult. Others had both pelvic and spinal deformities that required custom shaping of support surfaces to provide the necessary degree of control, support, and comfort. In general, parents, teachers, and clinicians were desperately in need of better tools and devices to manage this population of young people with disabilities.

Throughout the late '60s, '70s and into the '80s, the subspecialty of specialized seating and mobility developed largely as a result of the needs of this younger population. The design challenge has been to evolve assessment tools and commercial designs that can meet their diverse needs. Today there is a wide variety of seating systems and wheel-based alternatives as the result of a most productive period of design/development and multidisciplinary problem solving.

Children and young adults with minimal to severe physical involvement can now be accommodated by a growing array of commercial options.

The challenge that now presents itself is to develop the educational programs and evaluation tools to assist clinicians and consumers in selecting the seating and mobility combinations that are the most appropriate for the needs of a specific child and family. Also, experiences gained with this latter group, especially in upper body control, are now beginning to filter over to those with spinal cord injuries, whose seating devices have been limited largely to pressure-relief cushion technology.

More recently, other populations (such as elderly persons and those who have sustained traumatic brain injury) have presented new design and clinical challenges to those working in the seating and mobility field. It is estimated that the elderly population is by far the largest potential user of wheeled mobility and seating devices (Bardsley 1984).

Management of older persons in hospitals, nursing homes, and in the community often involves long periods of sitting. The traditional sling-type wheelchair meets few of the needs of this population, especially if their nonambulatory status is permanent. Lack of appropriate body support, formation of pressure sores, and general discomfort are significant remaining problems that are not well resolved by the technology services provided to this large group today (Shaw 1988).

Rehabilitation management of persons who have sustained a brain injury, the majority of which are young males, engenders another array of clinical and community requirements for seating and mobility technology. The early rehabilitation phase is often marked by rapid changes in a person's ability to control body movements and posture. Prevention of deformity that can result from asymmetrical muscle activity can be another requirement.

The need for independence in mobility can present a special challenge, especially when upper body function is severely affected and manual propulsion may or may not be a functional outcome. This is complicated by visual, cognitive, and perceptual deficits. Research designs and clinical solutions are just now beginning to develop. Prototype testing is evident in a number of development centers. The next few years should realize a number of vastly improved technological solutions for those with brain injuries.

Other Developments

Important ancillary developments are also taking place in the rehabilitation technology field. For example, tremendous growth has occurred in the support services necessary to deliver seating and mobility technology.

The organization of multidisciplinary teams, trial exemplary client flow models, development of evaluation and assessment tools, identification of new funding options, and experimentation with a variety of innovative regional, statewide, or provincial models for delivery of rehabilitation technology are all vitally important to the future growth of the field.

Parallel technological developments are also occurring rapidly. Developments in the field of augmentative communication devices, computer access interfaces, and environmental control systems are also increasing the functional levels of many people using specialized seating and mobility. Although these technologies are not the primary focus of this book, the integration of seating and mobility technologies with these other developments—in order to meet the comprehensive needs of people—is becoming an important clinical necessity.

And finally, tools for designers are emerging in the form of anthropometric data on those with disabilities and on performance standards for wheelchairs.

Philosophy of Dynamic Seating
and Independent Mobility

Scientific and Engineering Concepts

Engineers have become directly involved as members of rehabilitation teams only as recently as the mid-1960s. Most of the significant biomechanical research on specialized seating and mobility has occurred since that time. It should be stated at the onset that there remain many unanswered questions, much analysis to be undertaken, and quantitative methods to be developed.

Scientists and engineers are now just beginning to appreciate the scope and subtlety of clinical problems in this exciting new field. The following overview highlights the more recent research and development achievements that are pioneering the scientific and clinical knowledge contributed in specialized seating and mobility.

The Seated Posture

Ergonomists have studied the seated posture for many years (Grieco 1986). They have been concerned primarily with improving comfort and minimizing back pain due to poor postures imposed by the seated work place. Anthropometrists have measured the body dimensions in the seated posture, which has been particularly useful for furniture and automobile design (Diffrient, Tilley, and Bardagjy 1974; Snyder et al. 1977).

More recent work has been carried out to provide anthropometric data on people with disabilities (Hobson et al. 1987) and the elderly population (Molenbroek 1987), who have body measurement parameters that can vary significantly from the young able-bodied population.

A great deal of biomechanical analysis has been done on the spine, particularly as it relates to lower back pain and principles of surgical management. For example, early biomechanical analysis was done on the role of internal pressures of the abdominal cavity on support of the spine (Nachemson, Elfstrom, and Kenedi 1972). The intent was to analyze the forces related to specific activities and postures that cause the greatest forces within the spinal structures, which over time can cause disc rupture and chronic back pain (Anderson, Ortengren, and Nachemson 1980; Occhipinti et al. 1985).

Others have undertaken complete biomechanical modeling of the spine as a mechanical structure in an effort to analyze the forces acting on the various structures (Yetterman and Jackman 1980).

Spinal and Pelvic Deformity

Of greater interest to the field of specialized seating is the biomechanics of spinal and pelvic deformity. A large percentage of individuals who use specialized seating devices have spinal deformities.

Spinal deformities are described clinically by degrees or types of lateral/rotational curvature (scoliosis), forward flexion (kyphosis), or extension (lordosis) of the spinal column. Most deformities begin as "flexible curvatures," which means that the full range of normal motion can be obtained actively or through passive manipulation.

Through applications of asymmetrical loading over time, the skeletal and ligamental structures assume permanent structural changes which result in "fixed" deformities, denoted by the inability to obtain the normal range of motion. Little can be done to reverse a fixed spinal or pelvic deformity short of surgical intervention.

At present, the specialized seating devices can do little more than accommodate, support, or slow the progression of a deformity. The natural history of spinal deformity, which includes the pelvis, is dependent on the nature of the primary disability. In cerebral palsy, the prevalence and incidence of spinal deformity has been well documented (Madigan and Wallace 1981; Robson 1968; Rosenthal, Levine, and McCarver 1974).

21

Studies have been done in an effort to determine the muscle imbalance along the spinal column (Ford and Bagnall 1984). Clinical observation and several research studies have shown that body segment positioning can reduce abnormal muscle tone (Nwaobi 1986; Nwaobi et al. 1983).

The current seating approach in cerebral palsy is to minimize the effects of spasticity by placing children in appropriate seated posture. However, it remains scientifically unclear as to what effect this may have on preventing the development and progression of spinal deformity, since no longitudinal studies have been done with adequate control groups.

Surgical or orthotic intervention is an alternative form of spinal management. In general, surgery of the spine for children with cerebral palsy is uncommon, done only if absolutely necessary. Typically, spinal surgery involves extensive procedures. Postsurgical management can be complicated by the persistence of the spasticity.

Spinal orthoses have been attempted with children who have cerebral palsy, with mixed results. In general, conventional spinal orthoses are not tolerated well by nonambulatory children with cerebral palsy. A modified orthosis which incorporates the pelvis has been developed by Carlson and Winter (1978). This system, called the Sitting Support Orthosis (SSO), can help to level the pelvis and apply the necessary forces to the thorax to minimize the detrimental effects of gravity and spastic muscle activities.

For other children with disorders such as Duchenne muscular dystrophy, the progression of the disease and loss of trunk musculature typically results in gross scoliotic deformities, usually early in the second decade. Surgical intervention is becoming the management of preference for this population, although many do not opt for surgery and therefore spinal orthoses or specialized seating are the remaining alternatives (Silverman 1986).

Zackarkow (1984) and Drummond, Breed, and Narechania (1985) focus on the problem of spinal and pelvic deformities in the population with spinal cord injuries. In order to maintain anterior/posterior trunk balance in the posture imposed by the traditional wheelchair sling seats, a person slides the pelvis forward, with the spine assuming a long "C"-shaped (anteriorly flexed, kyphotic) position.

When higher spinal lesion levels are present, this posture can also include lateral flexion and rotation (scoliosis) of the spine. These deformities can contribute to an increase in pressure-related problems experienced by those with spinal cord injuries (Drummond, Breed, and Narechania 1985; Hobson and Nwaobi 1985).

Biomechanics of Deformity in the Seated Posture

Several clinical investigators describe the biomechanics of deformity in children with cerebral palsy in the seated posture. Nwaobi (1984) describes the alignment changes in the spine and pelvis that normally occur when going from standing to sitting. Also, the three-point lateral force system and the effect of tight hamstrings on tilt alignment of the pelvis are explained.

Carlson et al. (1986) emphasize the importance of leveling the pelvis in the frontal plane. They also illustrate the importance of the seat shape and its inclination in controlling pelvic alignment. Rang et al. (1981) discuss the biomechanics of common deformities encountered in seating children with cerebral palsy.

Letts et al. (1984) describe the relationship between spinal and pelvic deformities, outlining the factors associated with wind-swept hip deformity. This deformity, which involves the spine, pelvis, and hip joints, usually presents a difficult management problem in specialized seating.

A great deal of investigative study remains to be done on the effects of positioning on spinal deformity, especially in those with cerebral palsy. Also, additional biomechanical studies are urgently needed on the effects of external support in minimizing or reducing spinal deformity in all populations utilizing specialized seating systems.

Evaluation and Equipment Selection

The primary goal of seating and mobility applications is to maximize the function, comfort, and independence of those who must use the technology in their daily lives. Within this broad objective is the need to make appropriate equipment selections and modifications and to create designs that serve the unique needs of individual users.

As the number of commercial options increases, the complexity and importance of appropriate equipment selection and follow-up processes is becoming more evident. For many, evaluation of an individual's physical, functional, psychosocial, and environmental needs must be undertaken to ensure desired outcomes. Evaluation, goal setting, and service provision carried out within a multidisciplinary environment most often yield the desired results, especially for those with the more severe handicapping conditions.

Additionally, it is vital that consumers be informed as to the many options that exist so that they can make informed choices about the technology that will influence their daily lives.

In summary, the field of seating and mobility technology is a rapidly emerging subspecialty within the rehabilitation engineering/assistive technology field. The commercial availability of technical options has increased dramatically over the past decade. Today there are more than 20 specialized seating options.

The growth of mobility options has been equally phenomenal. At least 15 models of lightweight chairs of varied designs, complemented by an increasing number of new powered models with creative control options, have become available in recent years.

The challenge now is to make wise choices regarding the use of these exciting developments. A critical future step for the continued maturity of the field is the increased participation of knowledgeable consumers and clinicians working in multidisciplinary environments committed to the provision of quality services.

References

Anderson, G. B. J., R. Ortengren, and A. L. Nachemson. 1980. Analysis and measurement of the loads on the lumbar spine during work at a table. *Journal of Biomechanics* 13:15.

Antczak, J. M., and E. Snell. 1987. A universal wheelchair feedback controller. In *Proceedings, RESNA tenth annual conference*, 593-94. Washington, DC: RESNA Press.

Aylor, J. H., and S. H. Lim. 1987. Improvements and performance of an adaptive battery monitor. In *Proceedings, RESNA tenth annual conference*, 498-99. Washington, DC: RESNA Press.

Bardsley, G. I. 1984. The Dundee seating programme. *Physiotherapy* 70:59.

Brown, K. E., and R. M. Inigo. 1987. An adaptive microcomputer-based controller for electric wheelchairs. In *Proceedings, RESNA tenth annual conference*, 536-37. Washington, DC: RESNA Press.

Brubaker, C. E. 1986. Wheelchair prescription: An analysis of factors that affect mobility and performance. *Journal of Rehabilitation Research and Development* 23:19.

Brubaker, C. E., I. S. McClay, and C. A. McLaurin. 1984a. Effects of seat position on wheelchair propulsion efficiency. In *Proceedings, second international conference on rehabilitation engineering*, 12-14. Washington, DC: RESNA Press.

_____. 1984b. The effect of mechanical advantage on handrim propulsion efficiency. In *Proceedings, second international conference on rehabilitation engineering*, 15-16. Washington, DC: RESNA Press.

Brubaker, C. E., C. A. McLaurin, and I. S. McClay. 1985. A preliminary analysis of limb geometry and EMG activity for five lever placements. In *Proceedings, RESNA eighth annual conference*, 350-52. Washington, DC: RESNA Press.

_____. 1986. Effects of side slope on wheelchair performance. *Journal of Rehabilitation Research and Development* 23:55.

Carlson, J. M., J. Larsen, K. O. Beck, and D. C. Wilkie. 1986. Seating for children and young adults with cerebral palsy. *Clinical Prosthetics and Orthotics* 10:137.

Carlson, J. M., and R. Winter. 1978. The Gilette sitting orthosis. *Orthotics Prosthetics* 32:34.

Collins, T. G., and J. J. Kauzlarich. 1987. Analysis of parameters related to the directional stability of rear caster wheelchairs. In *Proceedings, RESNA tenth annual conference*, 507-9. Washington, DC: RESNA Press.

Diffrient, N., A. Tilley, and J. C. Bardagjy. 1974. *Human scale 1/2/3*. Cambridge, MA: Henry Dreyfuss Association.

Drummond, D., A. L. Breed, and R. Narechania. 1985. Relationship of spine deformity and pelvic obliquity on sitting pressure distributions and decubitus ulceration. *Journal of Pediatric Orthopedics* 5:396.

Everest, H. A., and H. C. Jennings. 1937. U.S. Patent 2,095,411.

Fisher, W. E., R. E. Garrett, and B. R. Seeger. 1988. Testing of gel-electrolyte batteries for wheelchairs. *Journal of Rehabilitation Research and Development* 25:27.

Ford, D. M., and K. M. Bagnall. 1984. Paraspinal muscle imbalance in adolescent idiopathic scoliosis. *Spine* 9.

Grieco, A. 1986. Sitting posture: An old problem and a new one. *Ergonomics* 29:345.

Hobson, D. A., and O. M. Nwaobi. 1985. The relationship between posture and ischial pressure for the high risk population. In *Proceedings, RESNA eighth annual conference*, 338-40. Washington, DC: RESNA Press.

Hobson, D. A., C. G. Shaw, L. C. Monahan, and C. McLarin. 1987. Anthropometric data for design of specialized seating and mobility devices—A preliminary report. In *Proceedings, RESNA tenth annual conference*, 338-40. Washington, DC: RESNA Press.

Inigo, R. M., and K. S. Kim. 1987. An energy-storage DC-DC converter for electric wheelchair drives. In *Proceedings, RESNA tenth annual conference*, 495-97. Washington, DC: RESNA Press.

Jagacinski, R. M., D. L. Hawthorne, D. S. Childress, R. van Vorhis, and J. Strysik. 1987. Using a time delay to alleviate oscillations with an electric wheelchair. In *Proceedings, RESNA tenth annual conference*, 492-94. Washington, DC: RESNA Press.

Johnson, B. W., J. H. Aylor, and R. D. Williams. 1987. The application of fault tolerance to microprocessor-based wheelchair control systems. In *Proceedings, RESNA tenth annual conference*, 784-86. Washington, DC: RESNA Press.

Kauzlarich, J. J., T. Bruning, and J. G. Thacker. 1983. Wheelchair caster shimmy and turning resistance. *Journal of Rehabilitation Research and Development* 20:15.

Kauzlarich, J. J., and B. C. Junkmann. 1987. A new battery with very long life for electric wheelchairs. In *Proceedings, RESNA tenth annual conference*, 501-3. Washington, DC: RESNA Press.

Kauzlarich, J. J., and J. G. Thacker. 1985. Wheelchair tire rolling resistance and fatigue. *Journal of Rehabilitation Research and Development* 22:25.

Kegel, B. 1985. *Journal of Rehabilitation Research and Development, Clinical Supplement* 1.

Letts, R. M., L. Shapiro, K. Mulder, and O. Klassen. 1984. The wind-blown hip syndrome in total body cerebral palsy. *Journal of Pediatric Orthopedics* 4(1).

Madigan, R., and S. Wallace. 1981. Scoliosis in the institutionalized cerebral palsy population. *Spine* 6.

McLaurin, C. A., and C. E. Brubaker. 1986. Lever drive system for wheelchairs. *Journal of Rehabilitation Research and Development* 23:52.

Molenbroek, J. F. M. 1987. Anthropometry of elderly people in the Netherlands; Research and applications. *Applied Ergonomics* 18:187.

Nachemson, A., G. Elfstrom, and R. M. Kenedi. 1972. Intravital measurement of forces in the human spine: Their clinical implication for low back pain and scoliosis. In *Proceedings, perspectives in biomedical engineering*, 111-19. Philadelphia: Lippincott.

Nwaobi, O. M. 1984. Biomechanics of seating. In *Seating for children with cerebral palsy—A resource manual,* edited by E. Trefler, 37-54. Memphis, TN: University of Tennessee.

———. 1986. Effects of body orientation in space on tonic muscle activity of patients with cerebral palsy. *Developmental Medicine and Child Neurology* 28:41.

Nwaobi, O. M., C. E. Brubaker, B. Cusick, and M. D. Sussman. 1983. Electromyographic investigation of extensor activity in cerebral palsied children in different seating positions. *Developmental Medicine and Child Neurology* 25:175.

Occhipinti, E., D. Colombini, C. Frigo, A. Pedotti, and A. Grieco. 1985. Sitting posture: Analysis of lumbar stresses with upper limbs supported. *Ergonomics* 28:1333.

Rang, M., G. Douglas, G. C. Bennet, and J. Koreska. 1981. Seating for children with cerebral palsy. *Journal of Pediatric Orthopedics* 1:279.

Reswick, J. B. 1985. Automatic transmission for electric wheelchairs. *Journal of Rehabilitation Research and Development* 22:42.

Robson, P. 1968. The prevalence of scoliosis in adolescents and young adults with cerebral palsy. *Developmental Medicine and Child Neurology* 10:447.

Rosenthal, R. K., D. B. Levine, and C. L. McCarver. 1974. The occurrence of scoliosis in cerebral palsy. *Developmental Medicine and Child Neurology* 16:664.

Seeger, B. R., and R. E. Luxton. 1984. A crashworthy restraint system for disabled people in wheelchairs in motor vehicles. In *Proceedings, second international conference on rehabilitation engineering,* 17-18. Washington, DC: RESNA Press.

Segner, S. E., and J. L. Bergstrand. 1987. A comparison of three-wheeled human powered bicycles for persons with physical disabilities. In *Proceedings, RESNA tenth annual conference,* 550-52. Washington, DC: RESNA Press.

Shaw, C. G. 1988. *Improved seating for the elderly—Project 1: Needs assessment. Final report.* Memphis, TN: University of Tennessee.

Sheth, P. N., and Brubaker, C. E. 1987. A spinal musculoskeletal model for wheelchair lever propulsion. In *Proceedings, RESNA tenth annual conference,* 486-488. Washington, DC: RESNA Press.

Shire, B. 1987. Microcomputer-based scanning interface for powered wheelchairs. In *Proceedings, RESNA tenth annual conference,* 541-43. Washington, DC: RESNA Press.

Silverman, E. 1986. Commercial options for positioning the client with muscular dystrophy. *Clinical Prosthetics and Orthotics* 10:159.

Smith, H. P. 1940. U.S. Patent 2,224,411.

Smith, R., I. Perkash, L. Leifer, D. Ives, D. Napolitano, and S. Shindell. 1984. Wheelchair feedback controller. *Rehabilitation R & D Progress Reports, vol. 3,* 151-57. Publication of the Rehabilitation Research and Development Service, Department of Medicine and Surgery, Veterans Administration, Washington, DC.

Snyder, R. G., L. W. Schneider, C. L. Owings, H. M. Reynolds, M. S. Golombdh, and M. A. Schork. 1977. *Anthropometry of infants, children, and youth to age 18* (sp. 450). Warrendale, PA: University of Michigan, Highway Safety Research Institute, Society of Automotive Engineers.

Taylor, S. 1986. A powered mobility evaluation system. In *Selected readings on powered mobility for children and adults with severe physical disabilities,* edited by E. Trefler, K. Kozole, and E. Snell, 69. Washington, DC: RESNA Press.

Trefler, E., and J. Marcrum. 1987. Trends in powered mobility for school aged physically handicapped children. In *Proceedings, RESNA tenth annual conference,* 510-13. Washington, DC: RESNA Press.

Trefler, E., J. Nickey, and D. A. Hobson. 1987. Technology in the education of multiply-handicapped children. *American Journal of Occupational Therapy* 37:381.

Verburg, G., D. Field, and S. Jarvis. 1987. Motor, perceptual, and cognitive factors that affect mobility control. In *Proceedings, RESNA tenth annual conference,* 468-70. Washington, DC: RESNA Press.

Wilson, A. B. 1986. *Wheelchairs—A prescription guide.* Charlottesville, VA: Rehabilitation Press.

Woude, L. H. V., H. E. J. Veeger, and R. H. Rozendal. 1987. Speed regulation in handrim wheelchair propulsion. In *Proceedings, RESNA tenth annual conference,* 483-85. Washington, DC: RESNA Press.

Yetterman, A. L., and M. J. Jackman. 1980. Equilibrium analysis for the forces in the human spinal column and its musculature. *Spine* 5.

Zackarkow, D. 1984. *Wheelchair posture and pressure sores.* Springfield, IL: Charles C. Thomas.

Powered Mobility: A Viable Option

Powered Mobility: A Viable Option

The importance of being independently mobile in one's environment cannot be overstated. Infants learn about their bodies and the space around them through movement. They begin their quest for independence by physically separating themselves from their parents. As children, they begin to use mobility devices such as scooters and bicycles to go further afield. Adults drive cars, fly on planes, and generally are as mobile in as large a sphere as is possible and affordable.

The degree to which mobility is important becomes even more apparent when noting the reluctance with which elderly persons give up driving in spite of their decline in perceptual, motor, and sensory faculties.

For persons with physical disabilities, movement—and in particular, independent movement—is just as important. Mobility technology should be utilized to supplement motor skills to accomplish this goal, yet for many, mobility devices are still considered a luxury or reward. This chapter presents the concept that mobility is a basic human right and that, whenever possible, mobility should be under the control of the individual. Later chapters on specific disabilities address specific concerns, with guidelines on evaluation and prescription for mobility technology.

Manual versus Powered Mobility

The first issue to be raised is whether a person needs manual mobility or powered mobility. (While manually operated wheelchairs can be operated either by an attendant or by the individual, this chapter will consider only self-propelled mobility.) If a person can efficiently operate a manual device within the environment, then a manual device is appropriate.

The environment in which a mobility device is to be used will vary with each person and may vary for an individual at different stages of life. A child of two would need to be mobile in the home, the classroom, and a very limited outdoor environment. As the child enters elementary school, the environment grows to encompass the school as a whole and a greater outdoor space, depending on whether the home is in an accessible neighborhood.

College widens the outdoor environment and, as adults, people want to be able to travel outside their immediate surroundings. The environment begins to shrink as the person ages. For the elderly who are homebound or in an extended-care facility, the need is for mobility within the facility and limited outdoor space.

Efficiency and Energy Demands

The other issue to be considered is efficiency. Independent mobility should not leave the person so exhausted that it becomes difficult for that person to perform other tasks. Children should be able to keep up with their peers. Young adults must be able to keep to a class schedule, and adults need to be able to work. All ages need a reservoir of energy to participate in recreational endeavors.

Deciding where one wishes to expend one's energy is a very individual matter, and professionals must be extremely careful not to dictate what is a reasonable environment to access for someone else. The person using the mobility device is the one to outline the needs.

Additionally, professionals must not confuse mobility with exercise. If an individual needs to lose weight or strengthen muscles, these need to be addressed in the context of therapy and carried out as part of a regular exercise or therapy program. To insist that a person use a manual chair to strengthen muscles or maintain respiratory capacity is not considered appropriate. Mobility is a basic right and should be as efficient and accessible as possible.

Mobility Concerns at
Different Life Stages

Children

Young children who are severely motor impaired often cannot move independently. This lack of movement severely limits their social, cognitive, perceptual, and functional development. By providing a means of independent mobility, many of the barriers to normal child development will be minimized.

Movement has been linked with the acquisition of cognitive skills in normal children (Campos and Bertenthal 1987). In addition, parents and therapists have supplied a great number of clinical stories about the increase in positive self-image and independence in play and activities of daily living, as well as a decrease in negative behaviors (such as crying or verbal manipulation) once children have received powered mobility devices.

Children become less dependent on verbally controlling their environment, more interested in all mobility skills including ambulation, and much more active in peer activities. Self-image is improved considerably, and attitudes toward approaching new tasks become more positive.

Traditionally, the time to consider powered mobility for persons with physical disabilities was as they entered adulthood. There were many reasons given to support this time-honored stand. Children, it was felt, did not need a powered wheelchair. Such equipment was too expensive and children were not sufficiently mature to respect this high-cost technical aid. It was felt that the walls of homes and schools were in jeopardy while children learned to direct battery-powered devices.

Families were told that transportation of powered chairs was difficult and purchase should be considered only if the family owned a van.

Therapists were adamant that children should never be given a powered wheelchair if they had any potential at all to propel a manual chair. The rationale was that children should be using their own motor abilities so they would remain functional. The only known exception was in the case of young adults with advanced muscular dystrophy.

Finally, it was felt that any child with any degree of mental retardation would never be capable of learning to operate and care for an expensive and complex technical aid.

The positive results of current research should be enough to change the attitudes of even the most skeptical professionals as more young children with severe disabilities are receiving powered mobility at earlier ages (Trefler and Marcrum 1988).

Over the last 20 years, research and clinical experience have shown that children starting at around 15 months of age are able to operate powered mobility devices safely (Butler, Okamoto, and McKay 1983; Paulson and Christofferson 1987). Even younger children are on prone scooters and adapted tricycles and are using motorized toys. Obviously, as with any young child, a training period and adult supervision are recommended.

Cost, transportation, and accessibility problems still exist. However, they can be overcome. Folding, lightweight chairs are now available. Physicians are writing letters to justify powered devices as being medically necessary for the child's overall development and welfare. Parents, especially once they see the positive effects of independent mobility, are becoming persistent in acquiring the devices.

Children, by nature, are inquisitive. They want to explore, misbehave, and run away when angry. How can they be children if they sit immobile in a wheelchair they cannot propel? How can they be taught a sense of responsibility when they must always depend on others for their daily tasks?

With advanced technology, even many of the most severely physically involved can potentially drive a powered chair. Innovative control systems are necessary, and not all bases are appropriate. However, it is the severely physically involved child who most needs the independence of mobility.

Ideally, powered systems should be provided to appropriate mobility impaired children as early as 24 months of age. If children must wait until they are older, many valuable years of learning are lost.

Independence and responsibility must be allowed and taught from an early age. The children learn not to hit walls. They learn to remember to ask someone to charge the batteries. They learn to go in straight lines and how to get out of tight corners. They learn how to be responsible for their own timetables at school. Given mobility, they experience movement and control. They can explore and they can run away. They can be children!

Adults

It is acknowledged that many adults require powered mobility to go to school or the workplace. However, it is often still a struggle to acquire the technology that can make working possible. Persons with high-level quadriplegia, persons with degenerative neuromotor problems, and even those with cerebral palsy do not automatically receive what they need.

Ongoing dialogue with insurance companies, worker's compensation programs, vocational rehabilitation, and the like, can delay or postpone acquisition of recommended technology. Even some in the medical community impose their biases and prevent acquisition because it is not, in their opinion, "necessary."

Elderly Persons

There has been a trend recently to provide senior adults with augmentative mobility devices (such as scooters) that are in broad usage for shopping excursions and other outings.

Against the resistance of staff and even some family members, residents in extended facilities are also being provided with powered mobility devices if they do not have the strength to propel a manual system. With the proper training and supervision, safety is not a major problem.

Within clinical circles, there is a growing body of anecdotal evidence on the benefits of powered mobility for this population. Clients who initially are very agitated and require considerable restraint show a marked decrease in the need for restraint, and their levels of agitation diminish, sometimes disappearing totally. Documentation verifies a decrease in agitation and negative behaviors when some control over personal mobility is returned to the individual (Bailey and Gilbert 1989).

Fortunately, attitudes about powered mobility are beginning to change. More children have access to powered devices (Trefler and Marcrum 1988), and more third-party payers are paying for them. With clinical research and documentation, more senior adults will have access to a variety of options.

Important Components in Providing Powered Mobility

Evaluation Equipment

Until every mobility clinic has some type of mobility evaluation technology, primitive methods will still be used to make decisions. Fortunately, there are now several powered chairs on the market that accept a variety of input devices (*Mobility Focus* 1992). These powered devices can accept an individual's own seating system, or an improved system can be simulated using commercial seating components (Taylor 1986).

Especially for persons with severe physical disabilities, an optimum seated position must be obtained *before* the individual is asked to perform the motor skills required to operate a switch(s), joystick, keypad, and so forth.

Another factor to consider is the ability to observe firsthand how the client responds to movement through space. There is a learning curve, and judgments must not be made too quickly. Training can provide the opportunity for clients to practice skills to gain a higher level of competence. Clinical experience has shown the importance of this step in the evaluation process that cannot be duplicated with computer simulation or anticipated through interview.

- A teenager with severe visual impairment was able to maneuver a complex obstacle course even though it had been predicted that she could not see well enough.

- A young male who was recovering from a head injury was able to operate a joystick with no problem. However, when he was placed in a powered device, he was unable to control his rage and tried to move full speed through a wall.

- Another person with a head injury was able to drive the chair safely but could not remember where he was.

- A young woman was able to develop perceptual skills to maneuver in very small spaces in spite of a communication system mounted in the only functional space—directly in her line of vision.

Experienced therapists have "gut feelings" when evaluating clients for mobility, sensing when skills will develop and when the family will persist until a functional level of competence is reached. But this is an insufficient basis on which to prescribe mobility devices, especially when thousands of dollars and individual freedom are at risk. Therapists and people with disabilities should insist on the use of functional evaluation equipment as a component of the evaluation process.

Evaluation Criteria

There are still few objective criteria which can guide clinicians in determining when a powered device is appropriate and safe. There are many complex issues. One research project has begun to determine cognitive predictors for successful control in very young children (Tefft, Furumasu, and Gueretta 1992). The project will also propose an approach for training. Although there are still more questions than answers, the questions must be raised.

Before persons can safely operate powered devices, they must have some understanding of cause and effect: "I move the stick or push the button, and the result is that I move."

There must also be some level of perceptual development, particularly spatial. Clients must be able to navigate through doorways and around furniture, and avoid steps and unramped curbs.

There must be a level of sensory processing. Clinicians have experience with persons with low vision who do just fine—but what of people who are blind? Can the use of high technology lasers be incorporated into powered device control to ensure safe operation?

There must also be a desire to move. This incorporates both a friendly environment and a desire to explore.

There does not yet exist a performance scale that reveals the IQ needed for a person to be a safe driver. The criteria for safe operation are so complex that IQ is unlikely to be the decisive factor. Children who are considered trainable but who have a strong desire to be mobile have been some of the safest and most responsible drivers. One boy of ten checked every night to see that his parents had examined the water level of the battery and had it charging for the next day. He knew that he wanted to be independent. To him, that meant his chair needed to be working.

Client Training

The availability of a comprehensive training component will often make the difference between equipment that is used and equipment that is stored. Few funding agencies will consider training in equipment purchase. People in rural areas cannot travel to the training facility. Either through home-, institution-, or community-based programs, sufficient training time (which will vary with the individual and the technology) must be provided.

In schools and in extended care and rehabilitation facilities, time can be scheduled as part of an ongoing therapy program. For persons in the community, more programs unique to their needs must be devised with caregivers becoming the primary trainers.

Funding

The funding of powered mobility technology, especially complex integrated systems, is still a challenge. But it is usually not impossible. Consumers, families, and professionals need to be more creative and persistent. Third-party payers, with justification, are paying for more systems that include powered wheelchairs. Some schools and institutions are, on a case-by-case basis, considering requests. Work-related recommendations are being considered. Families and friends are joining forces to approach religious institutions, industry, the business community, philanthropic groups, and others in fund-raising efforts. Many are successful.

A philosophical question remains. If professionals know that a person cannot afford an expensive solution, should that option be mentioned at all? The answer is *yes,* and the key word is *option.* Yes, the person/family needs to know about the best solution. They should also be informed about the other, more affordable options and the limitations these options may impose. Then they can make an informed choice.

The Team

While the composition of the team of people who work with a client will vary across the country, several factors should be constant. The client should hold the final decision-making responsibility. Professionals can evaluate, provide recommendations, help procure, and train. Professional expertise can be provided regarding functional abilities, safety issues, and reasonable expectations. However, it is the families or the individuals who must make the decisions. Do they want it? Can they transport it? Can it be accommodated into their lifestyle?

The team providing the client with sufficient information to enable them to make informed decisions can consist of a wide variety of people. Therapists, rehabilitation engineers, rehabilitation technologists, physicians, rehabilitation technology suppliers, and manufacturers often comprise the core group. The more complex the mobility technology and the more challenging the integration of other technologies (augmentative communication devices, environmental control systems, seating systems), the more highly trained and experienced the team. A therapist, alone in a rural school program, would most likely refer the student to a specialized team for evaluation although this person may do the training and provide valuable information to the evaluation and decision-making process.

Persons wanting to contact high technology centers could contact RESNA, an association for the advancement of rehabilitation technology (1101 Connecticut Ave. NW, Suite 700, Washington, DC 20036; 202/857-1199).

There is also a network in every state that is responsible for developing a statewide delivery system for technology. For information, contact the National Institute on Disability and Rehabilitation Research (NIDRR), U.S. Department of Education, 400 Maryland Ave. SW, Washington, DC 20202-2645 (202/732-5066).

Conclusion

The technology to provide almost every person who has a severe physical disability with appropriate mobility is available. There are many different options of manual and powered wheelchairs and bases. Controls vary from joystick to single switches to voice controls (Lee and Thomas 1990). Evaluation and training strategies must become more comprehensive and objective. Clinical research will help define decision-making criteria so that the client, the professional, and the payer will all feel confident in moving forward with independent mobility.

References

Bailey, J., and E. Gilbert. 1989. Mr. Crenna couldn't rest—and neither could we. *Nursing* November:50-51.

Butler, C., G. A. Okamoto, and T. M. McKay. 1983. Powered mobility for very young disabled children. *Developmental Medicine and Child Neurology* 25:472-74.

Campos, J. J., and B. I. Bertenthal. 1987. Locomotion and psychological development in infancy. In *Childhood powered mobility: Developmental, technical, and clinical perspectives.* In *Proceedings of first northwest RESNA regional conference,* 11-42. Washington, DC: RESNA Press.

Lee, K., and D. Thomas. 1990. *Control of computer-based technology for people with physical disabilities. An assessment manual.* Toronto, ON: University of Toronto Press.

Mobility Focus, a supplement to *Homecare,* June 1992 (*Homecare,* P.O. Box 16448, Hollywood, CA, 91615-6448).

Paulson, K., and M. Christofferson. 1987. Psychosocial aspects of technical aids—How does independent mobility affect the psychosocial development of children with physical disabilities? In *Proceedings, Second international conference of rehabilitation engineering,* 282-86. Washington, DC: RESNA Press.

Taylor, S. J. 1986. A powered mobility evaluation system. In *Selected readings on powered mobility for children and adults with severe physical disabilities,* edited by E. Trefler, K. Kozole, and E. Snell, 69-76. Washington, DC: RESNA Press.

Tefft, D., J. Furumasu, and P. Gueretta. 1992. Cognitive predictors of successful powered wheelchair control in very young children. In *Proceedings, RESNA international conference,* 412-13. Washington, DC: RESNA Press.

Trefler, E., and J. Marcrum. 1988. Trends in powered mobility for school aged physically handicapped children. In *Proceedings, Fourth international seating symposium, University of British Columbia,* 50-52. Vancouver, BC: University of British Columbia.

Biomechanics*

by Kevin Longfield, B.Sc., B.A.

*Reprinted by permission, Otto Bock, Canada

Biomechanics

"Mechanical science is the noblest and above all others the most useful . . . by means of it all animated bodies which have movement perform all their functions." Leonardo Da Vinci (Williams and Lissner 1969)

If a client is seated properly in a well-designed chair, comfort, quality of life, and health are all enhanced. If, on the other hand, the chair design is poor, or if the client is seated improperly, the client will not only be uncomfortable, but physical harm can result. A key component to providing clients with effective seating is an understanding of the forces acting on the human body.

This section explains the theories which form the basis of biomechanics, and how to apply those theories when seating individuals with a physical disability.

Mechanical science, or *mechanics,* is the study of forces and their effects on bodies. (In this context, a body is a physical entity, either solid, liquid, or gas.) *Biomechanics* relates forces in muscles, bones, and joints with externally-applied loads (Hobson 1983; Williams and Lissner 1969). The forces involved in biomechanics come from gravity, muscular action, and the resistance applied to body segments by other structures (Hobson 1983; Williams and Lissner 1969).

Definition of Force

While everyone has an intuitive understanding of what a force is, arriving at a concise scientific definition is difficult. A force tends to cause or prevent an action. It can be something easily detected and understood, such as a therapist pushing on a wheelchair to cause motion, or it can be something almost imperceptible, such as the gravitational attraction between a dust particle and a billiard ball. All forces, however, have certain traits in common (Hobson 1983; Williams and Lissner 1969):

1. Forces have magnitude. A person whose weight is 70 kilograms has a gravitational force of 70 kilograms acting on his or her body.

2. Forces have direction. The magnetic field of the earth draws a compass needle toward the North Pole.

3. Forces have orientation, or a line of action. They tend either to compress or extend the body they act upon. An accordion is played by continuously reversing the orientation of the force the hands apply to it.

4. Forces have a point of application. When a person sits erect on a flat surface, the force of gravity is applied to the chair largely through the ischial tuberosities. When the person stands, the soles of the feet absorb this force.

The study of mechanics is usually broken into two components: *statics* and *dynamics* (Hobson 1983; Williams and Lissner 1969). Statics involves forces acting upon a body at rest, and dynamics concerns itself with motion. Dynamics can be further subdivided into *kinematics* and *kinetics*. Kinematics describes motion without concern for the forces involved, while kinetics involves both the motion of the body and the forces acting upon it. The range of motions available to a body segment are determined through kinematics, but kinetics is used to determine the forces necessary to produce those motions.

When all of the forces acting on a body are balanced and no motion takes place, a state of *static equilibrium* exists. Static equilibrium is therefore a key objective in designing adaptive seating for a person with a disability. Adaptive seating is in many cases a replacement or supplement for muscular forces the person lacks. For instance, muscle tone provides resistance to gravitational forces in order to keep the spinal column erect. If muscle tone is lacking, however, spinal kyphosis will result unless the seating system provides corrective forces.

If, however, the forces are not balanced, motion occurs. If a therapist applies sufficient force to the handles of a wheelchair, the chair moves forward. If the forces acting on the chair are unbalanced, the chair will accelerate (change speed) in the direction of the greater force. If the chair moves at a constant velocity, however, it is said to be in a state of *dynamic equilibrium.*

It can be seen from the above that static equilibrium is really a special case of dynamic equilibrium: static equilibrium occurs when the body's velocity is constant at zero.

As was mentioned earlier, a body is the physical entity upon which a force acts. It can be either solid, liquid, or gas. In biomechanics, the human body is considered to be a solid body. For simplification, the body is usually considered to be rigid, so that the extent to which the applied forces deform the body are ignored, i.e., when considering the gravitational force acting on a client, the extent to which the bones compress as a result of this force is ignored.

Rigid body mechanics are governed by Newton's three laws of motion (Hobson 1983; Williams and Lissner 1969):

1. A body remains at rest or in uniform motion until acted upon by an unbalanced set of forces. This law is readily applied to a person sitting in a wheelchair. As was said earlier, balancing of forces is a key objective of adaptive seating. When adding a bolster or other support, care must be taken not to disturb the equilibrium of forces.

2. If an unbalanced force is applied to a body, the body's acceleration will be directly proportional to the force applied, and inversely proportional to the body's mass. (Force = mass times acceleration)

3. For every action, there is an equal and opposite reaction. When a body exerts a force on a second body, therefore, the second body exerts an equal but opposite force on the first body. When a bolster is applied to a patient's pelvis, the pelvis applies an equal and opposite force to the bolster. The bolster must therefore be able to withstand the force applied by the pelvis, and the force applied by the bolster must be applied in such a way that it causes no damage or discomfort to the client. This concern will be dealt with in greater detail later on.

As can be seen, the first and third laws are of particular importance in biomechanics.

Inertia
· ·

The first law is also known as the law of inertia. Inertia is defined as the tendency of bodies at rest to stay at rest, and the tendency of bodies in motion to stay in motion. Anyone who has pushed a stalled car has experienced both aspects of inertia: it takes a great deal of effort to get the car rolling, but it is also very difficult to stop the car once motion is achieved.

In adaptive seating, a state of static equilibrium is desired. It is often maintained by friction. The friction between the client's body and the seat cushion can help to maintain a seated posture in spite of gravitational and postural forces which tend to cause the client to slide out of the chair (Snijders 1988). Choice of cushion materials and contour is therefore an important factor in providing proper seating.

All posture and movement is influenced by the supporting surface; stepping onto a dance floor places a completely different level of demands upon the human body than stepping onto a skating rink.

Balance of Forces
· ·

Similarly, when designing an adaptive seating system, the caregiver must ensure that all applied forces and the reactions they cause are considered. Every force applied to the body has a reaction, and care must be taken to ensure that full consideration is given to the balance of forces. Improperly balanced forces can increase risk of injury by compromising stability, and they can cause damage by promoting deformity or tissue damage.

Balancing forces is a problem in statics. In balancing forces, special consideration must be given to *pressure*. Pressure is a measure of the effective area over which a force acts. It is defined as the total applied force divided by the area over which it acts. A block one meter square weighing ten kilograms exerts a pressure of ten kilograms per square meter on the surface upon which it rests.

Pressure is a vital consideration in a client's comfort. A person walking barefoot on a rocky beach experiences discomfort because the body's weight is borne by the sharp edges of the rocks. On the other hand, if the person wears walking shoes, the body's weight is spread over the surface of the soles, and discomfort is greatly reduced.

Similarly, a flat metal bolster will contact only a small portion of a client's body, as is shown in figure 10a. The entire corrective force will be transmitted to that area. The pressure on that area will be high, and therefore the probability of skin breakdown and pressure sores is increased. On the other hand, if the bolster is padded, and contoured to contact a greater body surface as in figure 10b, the pressure will be reduced and the corresponding comfort level increased (Cooper 1990, 1991).

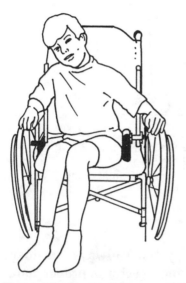 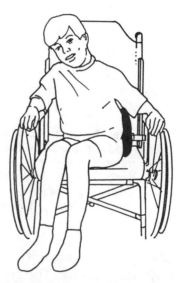

Figure 10a. Contact area against a flat bolster is small.

Figure 10b. A curved bolster gives a large support surface.

Analysis of Force Systems

In designing an adaptive seating system, careful analysis must be made of the forces which will act on the client. A valuable tool in this analysis is a graphical representation of the force system and the body it acts upon.

A force is considered a *vector* quantity (Hobson 1983; Williams and Lissner 1969), since it has magnitude and direction. A vector is a directed straight line, with a length proportional to the magnitude of the quantity, drawn in the direction the quantity acts. A vector is illustrated in figure 11. Force vectors are usually represented as arrows, with the head indicating the orientation or line of action of the force. The tail of the arrow attaches to the body under study at the point of application of the force.

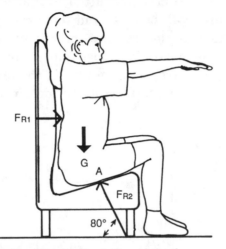

Figure 11. Vector representation of the force exerted on
the body by a seat cushion. On a scale of 1 cm = 20 Kg,
    magnitude = 40 Kg (arrow is 2 cm long)
    direction = 80 degrees from vertical in frontal plane
    point of application = A
    line of application is upward

Analysis of biomechanical force systems always considers gravitational forces. The gravitational vector is proportional to the weight of the body and is directed toward the center of the earth. A rigid body behaves as if the entire mass were applied to the body's center of gravity (Hobson 1983; Williams and Lissner 1969). (The center of gravity is the point in three-dimensional space about which the body is perfectly balanced; that is, any plane passing through the body at this point would divide it into halves of equal weight.) The point of application of the gravitational force is therefore the center of gravity.

Other forces do not necessarily act through the center of gravity. Forces which do not act through the center of gravity exert either shear forces or torque on the body.

Shear Forces (figure 12)

Shear forces act in opposite directions but are parallel to each other (Hobson 1983; Williams and Lissner 1969). As a client's body slides along a cushion, the skin experiences shear forces; the motion of the client's body is opposed by friction.

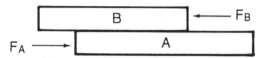

Figure 12. Shear forces. Forces F_A and F_B tend to push surfaces A and B apart.

Torque (figure 13)

Torque is the result of two opposing forces acting about an axis or pivot point which is perpendicular to the plane of the force (Hobson 1983; Williams and Lissner 1969). These forces (often called a couple) tend to cause rotation of the body and are said to exert a torque or moment about the body. An example of a moment in adaptive seating is the forces acting on the pelvis in asymmetrical seating. The gravitational force acts through the center of gravity, but since the body's weight is borne by only the lower ischial tuberosity, parallel opposing forces result, creating a moment. The resulting moment tends to rotate the pelvis in the frontal plane.

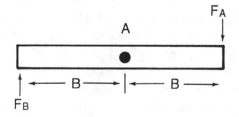

Figure 13. Torque. F_A and F_B exert torque about pivot point A. They each are of magnitude F and distance B from the pivot point, and therefore exert a clockwise moment of FxB on A. Such forces are called a couple.

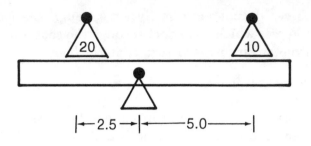

Figure 14. A large force and a small moment arm can balance a small force and a large moment arm.

A moment has two components: the magnitude of the force and the distance from the point of application to the pivot point. A moment's magnitude is therefore expressed in units of force and distance, such as Newton-meters or inch-pounds. Thus a small force acting over a great distance can have an equal effect to that of a large force acting over a small distance, as is illustrated in figure 14. Children playing on a teeter-totter make use of this principle to achieve equilibrium. This aspect of moments has enormous implications for adaptive seating, as is explained later in the chapter.

Analysis of Complex Force Systems

In real-life situations, the forces acting upon a client are often complex. Not all quantities are known when the analysis begins. Two general statics problems are used to resolve general force systems (Hobson 1983; Williams and Lissner 1969):

1. *Finding the resultant.* The analyst finds the simplest force or system of forces which will replace the more complex system. Often this is a single force or moment. For example, to determine the load applied to a vertebra when a person carries a weight in each hand, the resultant is the sum of the two weights and the weight of the person's body above the vertebra.

2. *Solving the equilibrium problem.* Newton's third law tells us that for every action there is an equal and opposite reaction. Solving the equilibrium problem takes

advantage of this law by working with the known quantities and using this information to solve for the unknown quantities. Knowing a client's weight helps us to determine the reactive forces to be absorbed by the wheelchair components.

Composition and Resolution of Forces

Composition entails adding forces to determine their net effect. The vectors of these forces are added, and the resultant force is determined from this sum. Remember that a vector has both magnitude and direction, so that the sum of two vectors is not just the arithmetic addition of the two magnitudes. Composition of two vectors is shown in figure 15.

Resolution of two forces is the opposite of composition. In this case the resultant force is known and is broken into its components. Figure 16 shows an example of resolution of forces. A client leaning on a bolster exerts both a horizontal and a vertical force on the part. Both components need to be known when determining the part's strength requirements.

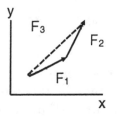

Figure 15. Composition of forces. Forces F_1 and F_2 combine to produce F_3.

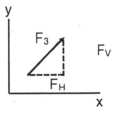

Figure 16. Resolution of forces. F_3 is made up of a horizontal component, F_H, and a vertical component, F_V.

Clinical Application of Biomechanical Principles in Seating

The challenge in seating the disabled population is similar to that of seating the normal population; the body supports must allow comfort and function for long periods (Snijders 1988). Adaptive seating must help the individuals with seating disabilities obtain seating which allows them to achieve the highest possible level of comfort, support, and function. Included in this goal may be any of the following objectives (Cooper 1990, 1991):

1. Increase stability
2. Improve orientation
3. Increase function
4. Improve appearance
5. Improve comfort

The limiting factors are biomechanics and the human body's ability to tolerate supportive forces and the associated pressure on body segments.

General Biomechanical Principles

Stability
· ·

The gravitational force acts through a body's center of gravity, so to stay upright, the gravitational vector must pass through the body's base of support. When standing, the base of support is the soles of the feet. If a person leans too far to one side, the center of gravity shifts outside the base of support, and a fall results. If the person senses that stability is about to be lost, one or both of the feet are shifted to move the center of gravity back inside the base of support.

In adaptive seating, stability must be achieved in two respects: the client must achieve a stable posture in the seating system, and the system itself must be stable.

The base of support for a seated person is the pelvis. The task in providing a stable posture is to provide a seat and back which will allow a stable pelvic position. With a stable base of support, a client's freedom of movement is enhanced. Asymmetrical seating and other abnormal seating postures can substantially decrease the size of the base of support, with a corresponding decrease in stability.

Friction between the client's body and the seat cushions helps the client to maintain posture. Cushion materials and shapes should be chosen with this fact in mind.

Providing a stable posture in a seating system is of little value, however, unless the seating system itself is stable. The system's base of support is the wheels. Increasing the wheelbase increases the base of support. Since gravity acts through the center of gravity, the client's center of gravity must be considered when designing a seating system. Generally, women have a lower center of gravity than men, and adults have a lower center of gravity than children. Changes in body structure, such as amputation or deformity, will also affect the center of gravity.

For maximum stability, the client's center of gravity should pass through the base of support and be as low as possible. The client's range of movements should also be considered. Placing the center of gravity too far forward can cause instability if the client leans forward, since leaning forward could shift the center of gravity outside the base of support. Seating the client too far to the rear can cause similar problems.

Lateral stability is also important. A wide wheelbase enhances lateral stability. In cases where deformity or other problems create habitual leaning to one side, stability is often enhanced by placing weights on the base of the other side to counterbalance the client's body.

Biomechanical Limitations

Pads and other seating components do not generate forces but supply the equal and opposite reactions to gravitational and muscle forces specified by Newton's third law (Cooper 1991). In blocking movement, the pads provide the point of application of the gravitational and muscular forces. The

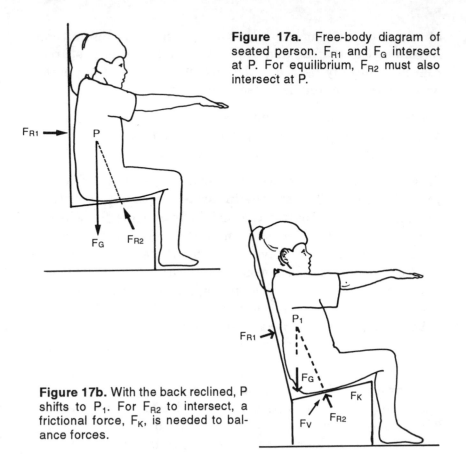

Figure 17a. Free-body diagram of seated person. F_{R1} and F_G intersect at P. For equilibrium, F_{R2} must also intersect at P.

Figure 17b. With the back reclined, P shifts to P_1. For F_{R2} to intersect, a frictional force, F_K, is needed to balance forces.

client's body specifies the magnitude, direction, and line of action of these forces. This is a major limitation in postural control.

A free-body diagram of a seated individual demonstrates the reactive forces involved (Snijders 1988). The reactive force on the back cushion and the gravitational force intersect at point P (figure 17a). For static equilibrium, the force of the seat cushion on the trunk must also pass through P. This force (and therefore the seat cushion) must therefore slope backwards slightly. If the back cushion reclines, however, as in figure 17b, a frictional force (the horizontal component of the force exerted on the trunk by the seat cushion) is needed to maintain equilibrium. This frictional force applies shear forces to the skin and underlying tissue, which will cause discomfort and damage if the shear forces are allowed to act long enough.

If both the seat and back are tilted at the same time, however, these shear forces vanish. The best seating systems for most clients, therefore, are those which maintain a constant seat-to-back angle of slightly greater than 90 degrees, regardless of the system tilt.

Pressure

Pressure is a major cause of discomfort and tissue damage; under normal conditions, skin breakdown is likely to occur if pressure exceeds two pounds per square inch. Pressure is a function of force and area, so positioning of pads and other supporting devices is crucial to reducing moment arms and therefore the reactive forces acting on the client's body. Frequently anatomical and other considerations dictate the pad positioning, and the only degree of freedom remaining to the seating specialist is the area of application.

Increasing the pad size will cause a commensurate decrease in pressure. Contouring will also increase contact area. Stability is enhanced with angled rather than curved surfaces, as it is easier for the body to slip around a curve (Cooper 1990). Angling the pad orientation will also increase contact area.

Controlling Movement about a Joint

Movement must be blocked on both sides of a joint to control orientation of a limb segment (Cooper 1990, 1991). Three forces must therefore be applied to the segment, as is shown in figure 18. Two forces immobilize the segment on one side of the joint, and the other force resists movement of the limb. This procedure is called three-point loading (Cooper 1990, 1991; Hobson 1983; Williams and Lissner 1969).

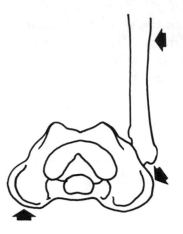

Figure 18. Three-point loading to correct hip abduction.

Maximizing Lever Length

The required holding force on the limb is influenced by the distance of the pad (reactive force) from the axis of rotation. The greater the distance, that is, the greater the moment arm, the lower the necessary holding force. Reducing the holding force reduces the pressure on the client's skin and underlying tissue. In the hip abduction example in figure 18, the holding force is doubled by moving the pad halfway down the femur toward the hip joint.

Choosing Pad Materials

Firm padding is more effective in maintaining posture than soft materials (Cooper 1990, 1991). Similarly, flexible components such as shoulder straps and lap belts, which depend upon the client to define their shape, do not maintain posture as well as rigid shoulder pads and pelvic bars. Since rigid materials may not provide as large an area of application as flexible materials, however, they may cause unacceptably high pressure concentrations. In these cases a flexible material may be preferable.

Seating Considerations

General

. . . .

Positioning is important in postural control. Sometimes even small body movements relative to the pad will severely compromise the pad's effectiveness. A secure, stable posture is therefore essential if the goals of the seating system design are to be met.

In seating, much of the body's stability comes from secure pelvic positioning (Carlson et al. 1986). Figure 19 shows the effect of a secure pelvis on trunk stability: a spinal column with an uncontrolled pelvis is similar to a flexible column jointed at its lower end. If, however, the pelvis is controlled (either by pads, belts, or a custom-contoured seat), the spinal column approximates a flexible column with a built-in base.

Buckling equations for elastic columns tell us that the built-in beam will withstand almost twice the load that the jointed column will before buckling (Carlson et al. 1986). Translated into seating terms, providing stable pelvic support makes it much easier to position the trunk in as upright a position as the client can tolerate. A *Cobb angle* reduction of almost 50% has been observed in X-rays of clients with flexible deformity seated with secure pelvic positioning (Carlson et al. 1986).

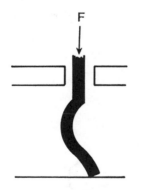

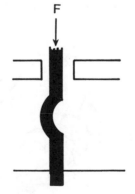

Figure 19a. A spinal column with an uncontrolled pelvis behaves like a flexible column jointed at the lower end.

Figure 19b. A spinal column with a controlled pelvis behaves like a column with a built-in base.

In controlling postural pelvic tilt (figure 20), two moments must be stopped: a posterior rotation of the top of the pelvis, and anterior rotation of the bottom (Cooper 1990, 1991). A firm back cushion will stop the top rotation, but stopping the anterior rotation is more difficult due to the lack of skeletal projections. Following are some of the alternatives:

Pelvic straps and subASIS bars
These block high on the pelvis but under the ASIS, and therefore have a short moment arm, with the resultant high reactive forces and pressures.

Anti-thrust blocks
Since these act on the ischial tuberosities, they offer a long moment arm. The disadvantage is that it is easy for the client to slip up and out of the blocks. The pelvis must therefore be held down by either a belt or bar.

Knee blocks
These are effective, but the client must have intact hip joints and symmetric tone about the pelvis.

Pommel stabilizers
These are controversial, but if installed and adjusted properly, they provide effective control. In conjunction with a lap belt they can inhibit tone, making a wide-base seating posture possible. Pommels should not be used as a means of preventing clients from sliding out of their seats.

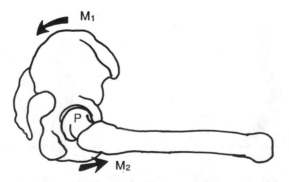

Figure 20. Posterior pelvic tilt. M_1 causes posterior rotation of top of pelvis about hip joint P. M_2 causes anterior rotation of bottom of pelvis about hip joint P.

Pelvic Obliquity and Rotation *(Cooper 1990, 1991)*

For obliquity, the caregiver must block elevation on one side and depression on the other. For rotation, anterior movement must be blocked on one side and posterior on the other.

Single pelvic belts are often ineffective against these conditions. If fitted very snugly, "Y" belts that trap the ASIS can be effective in controlling obliquity and rotation. Pommel stabilizers are completely ineffective because they lack a moment arm in this application. Anti-thrust bars have a good mechanical advantage against rotation and can work well in this application. A subASIS bar that blocks at the widest part of the pelvis is another possible solution for this application.

Wind-Swept Hips *(Cooper 1990, 1991)*

The three-point loading shown in figure 18 is required to correct wind-swept hips. Lateral pelvic control is also needed. Care must be taken not to introduce rotation of the trunk when positioning the knees; one solution is often a neutral shoulder and trunk position with the client's face looking forward, and with the knees being allowed to position laterally. Obliquity, scoliosis, and hip rotation often accompany wind-swept hips, complicating the seating design.

Scoliosis *(Cooper 1990, 1991)*

Support systems for scoliosis will not cure the condition; at best they will slow the progress of the scoliotic curve. "Correction" in this context means providing temporary support to enable the clients to assume a more upright posture.

Figure 21 shows the three-point loading used in scoliosis. Gravity exerts a large downward force which must be considered with the scoliosis forces in treating the problem. Straightening the trunk allows it to support the upper body weight better, and therefore the client's function is increased. Complete straightening is possible only with slight curvatures, however.

With greater curvatures the pads provide both gravitational and corrective support. Furthermore, the possible vertical separation of the pads is reduced, increasing the reactive force and therefore the pressure.

Sometimes the high side of the pelvis is left unsupported in the hope that gravity will supply a corrective force (Cooper 1990, 1991). This tactic is effective only for small obliquities; as the curvature increases, the gravitational moment arm decreases and becomes less effective.

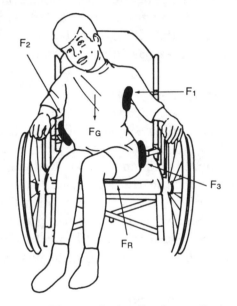

Figure 21. Three-point loading for scoliosis.

Internal Hip Rotation (Cooper 1990, 1991)

The three-point loading is applied medial at the knee, and lateral at the pelvis and lower leg. By blocking at the ankle or foot, a large corrective force is possible, due to the long moment arm. In some cases this force can be large enough to pose a risk of injury to the hip. In these cases the moment arm should be reduced by moving the pad closer to the hip joint.

Trunk Extension *(Cooper 1990, 1991)*
. . . .

The three-point loading is applied anterior to the pelvis and shoulders (remember that pads are preferable to belts) and posterior to the lumbar area. The posterior force is applied either to a flat seat back or lumbar pad. When a lumbar pad is used, often little separation exists between the lumbar pad and the anterior pelvic support. For this reason, anti-thrust blocks or knee blocks frequently accompany lumbar pads.

Sitting in Bed *(Snijders 1988)*
. . . .

Bed-ridden clients can be given a forward field of vision by tilting the head end of the bed to approximate a seating posture.

While this posture greatly enhances the quality of life, it poses certain problems:

- The pelvis rests on the coccyx instead of the ischia. The coccyx is much more sensitive.
- Friction between the skin and the bed, necessary to prevent the client from sliding off the end of the bed, causes shear forces.
- Eventually the client will slide forward, causing the clothes to wrinkle and underwear to gather at the crotch.

Foot blocks which bridge the gap between the feet and the end of the bed will help to reduce the friction and sliding problems. Another solution is to adjust the mattress so the knees and hips are bent. This mattress shape provides a barrier to sliding.

Conclusion

A sound knowledge of biomechanics is essential in designing seating for the disabled. Proper pad positioning can greatly increase client comfort and at the same time increase the therapeutic value of the system. Biomechanics is equally important in seating a disabled person. Sometimes even a small shift in body position relative to a pad can completely alter the usefulness of the seating system. The challenge for health care professionals is to provide a seating system that maximizes comfort, function, appearance, and therapeutic value.

References

Carlson, J. M., J. Lonstein, K. O. Beck, and D. C. Wilkie. 1986. Seating for children and young adults with cerebral palsy. *Clinical Prosthetics and Orthotics* 10(4):138-49.

Cooper, D. 1990 (February). Biomechanics in posture control. In *Proceedings, Sixth international seating symposium*, 32-38. Vancouver, BC: University of British Columbia.

_____. 1991 (February). Biomechanics of selected posture control methods. In *Proceedings, Seventh international seating symposium*, 37-40. Memphis, TN: University of Tennessee.

Hobson, D. A. 1983. Biomechanical concepts of specialized seating. In *AAOP seating symposium proceedings*, November 12-13. Chicago: AAOP.

Snijders, C. J. 1988. Design criteria for seating based on biomechanics. In *ICAART 88 Proceedings*, 472-73. Montreal, Quebec: ICAART.

Williams, M., and H. R. Lissner. 1969. *Biomechanics of human motion.* Philadelphia: W. B. Saunders.

. . . .

PART II

Evaluation and Prescription Principles and Practices

Principles of Evaluation

Cerebral Palsy

Head Injuries

Muscular Dystrophy

Spinal Cord

Elderly Clients

Principles of Evaluation

Principles of Evaluation

The Evaluation Process

The evaluation for assistive technology should include consideration of all functional needs of the individual and the possible technical devices that might be of assistance. In this book, the evaluation process will stress considerations for seating and mobility devices.

In many cases, a client might benefit from other technical devices such as prone standers or augmentative communication systems. These will be mentioned, particularly in relation to accessing multiple switch-operated devices, but will not be covered in any detail. The underlying premise is that dynamic, therapeutic seating will enhance the client's ability to access other devices in addition to helping the client be more comfortable and able to sit for longer periods.

Evaluations for seating and mobility are most effective when performed by a team of knowledgeable professionals with strong participation by the client. Not all therapists or physicians have the specific expertise to participate in the seating team. Additional training or apprenticeship is often necessary in order to have current information in seating practices and technology. Clients should look at not only the professional qualifications of the seating team, but their experience in the specific area of seating and mobility as well.

The UTREP Model

UTREP (the University of Tennessee Rehabilitation Engineering Program) is an outpatient clinic in a university structure. The team consists of a physician (orthopedic surgeon), therapists, engineers, a clinic coordinator, the client, and the primary caregiver. Because UTREP is an outpatient, university-based clinic, the client's therapists, counselors, and/or teachers are encouraged to participate in the evaluation process either in person or by sending their own written recommendations. Other models for technology delivery include inpatient services, private practice, and others (RESNA 1987).

The morning of the clinic is reserved for client screenings and evaluations by the therapy and engineering staff. Each client is scheduled for a one-hour seating/mobility evaluation. If the information received from the referring source indicates that the client needs a more intensive evaluation, then two hours may be scheduled. This might be the case with someone who has an acute head injury, when a client needs an opportunity to try powered mobility, or when a client has severe orthopedic deformities and breathing problems.

The client who needs more than two hours may require a complex powered mobility evaluation or an augmentative communication evaluation. In such cases, the evaluations often are scheduled on a day prior to the clinic.

When clients arrive, they are met by the client coordinator who ensures that all paperwork is complete (including medical records, funding information, and photo and liability releases). Front and side photographs are taken.

After the appropriate database is acquired, the therapist begins the evaluation, using the standardized Technical Aid Evaluation Form included at the end of this chapter (pages 76-83). Components of the evaluation include the neuromotor status, orthopedic condition, functional abilities, and psychosocial and environmental issues.

Based on information obtained by the therapist through interview and physical manipulation, a preliminary solution to the seating and mobility needs of the client is identified. A seating simulator is used to verify these conclusions by actually trying the position in possible systems. The simulator also provides the family and client with the ability to see the client in the new position.

Finally, measurements are taken from the simulator to assist with accurate fabrication at a later date. At this time, photographs are taken both for funding purposes and for a visual record for staff of the simulated seating position that worked well during the evaluation. If the technical needs are complicated, requiring customization of components, then an engineer will be included in the evaluation. Once the needs are identified, the client coordinator is able to speak to the family about possible funding for the proposed technology.

The actual clinic is held in the afternoon. During the clinic team meeting, at which the client is present, each professional's assessment is presented to the physician, who physically examines the client to determine if the recommendations are compatible with the general medical condition. Following a consensus on the type of technology to use, a prescription for equipment is generated or, as in the case of augmentative communication needs or complex powered mobility needs, a recommendation for a more in-depth evaluation is made.

Long-range goals for the client and the compatibility of the technical aids which are recommended must be considered during the prescription process. The team must plan for smooth implementation of each aspect of the client's technological needs over time. This ensures a functional and more cost-effective result. For example, it is more efficient to project the need for powered mobility at the time of the initial evaluation—even if the powered wheelchair will not be needed for another year—than to go back to the funding source six months after the purchase of a manual wheelchair and ask for a second, more costly, item which, to the uninformed, seems to fulfill a similar need.

If two wheelchairs are discussed during the initial evaluation, then any seating system prescribed must be fabricated to fit into both manual and powered chairs. Also, if the client must operate a communication device as well as a powered wheelchair, the control locations must be considered at the same time so as to offer optimum placement to both without functional compromise.

The setting of priorities should also be considered in relation to the client's overall need for services. Very young children can be seated in adaptive strollers. However, as soon as a child approaches school age, he or she must be in a wheelchair or other base that has a federally approved bus tie-down system. This need must be anticipated if the child is not to be excluded from school transportation systems.

With the adult population and children needing powered wheelchairs, their mobility needs are linked to both personal vehicle needs and community mobility needs. Vans with lifts are needed for transportation. Often vans require custom modification to permit comfortable and safe transportation.

Priorities should also include the need for other devices. If funding is a problem, which device should be procured first, the seating, the powered wheelchair, the augmentative communication device, or the computer? Establishing these priorities will vary from client to client depending on many individual circumstances. It is essential that the seating team not work in isolation, or many costly errors will be made.

Once the client is seen in the clinic, the initial evaluation phase is complete. A prescription for the technology is generated as well as a medical note for the records. The clinic coordinator then begins the search for the funding necessary to provide the technical devices recommended.

If a further, more in-depth evaluation is needed, that is scheduled and prescription is delayed until after the additional evaluation, to incorporate its findings. Usually, the physician does not see the client again but includes the therapist's verbal summary of the in-depth evaluation results in the notes and prescription.

Although the initial evaluation is complete, the therapists will reevaluate the clients each time they come for review or technical services. At such time as the medical condition, size, or functional needs change sufficiently to warrant a new system, the therapist will schedule the client for a clinic visit, and the process will be repeated.

At UTREP, therapists have the authority to make any repairs or modifications for growth, as well as system changes to accommodate to functional changes. It is only when a totally new system is required that the client is seen again by the physician.

Evaluation Tools

Simulators
. . . .

During the evaluation, seating and mobility simulators are used to determine optimal positions and potential or real functional abilities. In the past, evaluating a client for a seating system involved a great deal of speculation as to exactly what components to use, in what combination to provide them, and in what exact positions to mount them.

Within the past 15 years, prototype seating simulators for both planar and custom seating have been developed at UTREP and have proven to be very useful tools. Several models are now commercially available. The therapist can evaluate the client in the system, alter angles of the seat to the back, try varying positions in space, and determine component sizes and accessories that are required before making recommendations for a particular system.

Both parents and consumers can be shown the value of the seating system, a method that is much more effective than verbally speculating on how posture and function may improve. Technical information (such as mounting angles, thigh lengths, etc.) can be communicated to technicians directly from the simulator rather than through the evaluator. This results in fewer errors from misunderstandings during the fabrication process.

A simulator can provide custom positioning for children or adults who do not yet have their own seating systems for a switch-access evaluation leading to controlling a powered wheelchair, computer, or augmentative communication device. With added proximal stability provided by the seating, clients often can use their hands and heads for control when previous attempts were less successful.

Photographs of the client actually seated in the appropriate positioning device are helpful in demonstrating the importance of seating to third-party payers. Although the initial cost of purchasing a simulator for a seating clinic may seem to be high, it has been found over the years that the savings in evaluation time and fabrication time far outweigh the initial costs incurred.

Pressure Measurement Devices
. . . .

Pressure measurement devices are another essential evaluation tool for a seating program. These can be simple and inexpensive or complex and very costly. Several commercial units are available and should be used for all clients with insensitive tissues. Additionally, they can be very useful for clients experiencing discomfort or when strong forces are required to accomplish a seating goal. Monitoring pressure over time can help ensure a safe seating posture.

Pressure measurement devices are discussed in greater detail in Appendix B, Technology Overview (pages 257-293).

Evaluation by Diagnosis

It is not the intent of this book to provide the full scope of medical information related to each of the disabilities discussed. However, in the chapters that follow, there is a very brief introduction for each specific disability, then those medical issues which would directly affect the prescription for seating and mobility devices are addressed.

The evaluation process, regardless of disability, follows the format of the evaluation form developed at the University of Tennessee Rehabilitation Engineering Program. The seating/mobility evaluation consists of screening in areas of function and dysfunction including neuromotor status, orthopedic involvement, sensory status, muscle strength, functional abilities and ADL skills, environmental concerns, and psychosocial considerations.

Reference

RESNA. 1987. *Rehabilitation technology service delivery—A practical guide.* Washington, DC.

Technical Aid Evaluation Form

Name _____ Date of Birth _____

Diagnosis _____

Reason for Referral

1. Seating   2. Mobility   3. Communication   4. Other

Medical History

Recent surgeries: ☐ Yes   ☐ No

_____

Significant medical problems: ☐ Yes   ☐ No

_____

Neuromotor Summary

Obvious pathological reflexes:

☐ Asymmetric Tonic Neck Reflex   ☐ Symmetric Tonic Neck Reflex

☐ Tonic Labyrinthine Reflex—Supine   ☐ Tonic Labyrinthine Reflex—Prone

☐ Extensor Thrust   ☐ Positive Supporting

Which predominate in sitting? _____

Extremity tone
(Note: hypotonic, hypertonic, athetoid, ataxic, other with mild, moderate, or severe on the following:)

	Left	Right
Upper Extremities		
Lower Extremities		
Trunk		

Orthopedic Summary

Pertinent limitations in movement? ☐ Yes ☐ No
Orthopedic problems being followed? ☐ Yes ☐ No

Indicate *mild, moderate,* or *severe* on the following:

Spine:	Scoliosis	Kyphosis	Lordosis

Pelvis:	Rotation	Tilt

Lower Extremities: _____
Upper Extremities: _____
Head: _____
Comments: _____

© 1993 by The University of Tennessee, Memphis
Published by Therapy Skill Builders, a division of Communication Skill Builders, Inc. / 602-323-7500
This page may be reproduced for administrative use. (Catalog No. 4726)

Sensation

Intact: ☐ Yes ☐ No
Impaired: ☐ Yes ☐ No
Absent: ☐ Yes ☐ No

History of pressure sores? ☐ Yes ☐ No

Active sore(s) presently? ☐ Yes ☐ No

Where? _____

Any other pressure considerations? _____

Functional Summary

Relevant problems with strength: _____

_____

_____

Gross motor skills

Head control _____

Trunk control _____

Rolls _____

Scoots _____

Sits _____

Crawls _____

Stands _____

Walks _____

Fine motor skills

Hand dominance   R / L

Activities of daily living	Independent	Independent Assisted	Dependent	Equipment used
Dressing				
Feeding				
Bathing				
Toileting				
Transfers				
Mobility				
Housekeeping				

Comments: _____

_____

Communication Skills

Receptive level _____

Expressive level _____

Present means of communication

☐ none
☐ gestures
☐ facials
☐ signs

☐ vocals
☐ speech
☐ picture board
☐ symbol board

☐ alpha board
☐ word board
☐ writing/drawing
☐ typing

☐ electronic communication

Type of electronic aid: _____

Access to aid: _____

Interest in surroundings: _____

Response to environment: _____

Education/Work History

School/Place of employment: _____

Type of job: _____

Education level:

☐ Below grade level: _____

☐ Nonacademic _____

☐ Academic _____

☐ Grade level _____

Transcription available:

☐ car ☐ van ☐ van/lift ☐ bus ☐ bus/lift ☐ other

Lift type: _____

Accessibility into and within building: _____

Personal Summary

Home environment

Type of setting: ☐ rural ☐ suburban ☐ urban

Sidewalks? ☐ Yes ☐ No   Paved roads? ☐ Yes ☐ No   Indoor plumbing? ☐ Yes ☐ No

Accessibility into and within home: _____

Widest door (in inches): _____   Narrowest door (in inches): _____

Transportation available

☐ car ☐ van ☐ van/lift ☐ van/ramp

Car size: _____

Lift type: _____

Comments: _____

Goals of Seating

Pelvis _____

Lower extremities _____

Trunk _____

Head _____

Upper extremities _____

Orientation in space _____

Comments: _____

Overall Goals of Seating

(Select the two or three *highest* priorities)

1. Comfort for client
2. Decrease tone/reflexes
3. Ease of transporting
4. Pressure relief
5. Positioning for functional skills
6. Accommodate for deformities
7. Provide correction for orthopedic deformities

Other Technical Aids

Communication _____

Powered mobility _____

Other _____

Growth adjustments necessary? _____

Any allergies? _____
_____

Developed by Elaine Trefler, M.Ed., OTR, Susan Johnson Taylor, OTR/L, and the University of Tennessee Rehabilitation Engineering Program.

Cerebral Palsy

Cerebral Palsy

Cerebral palsy is a motor disorder caused by damage to or dysfunction of the immature brain. It is classified according to movement disorders and limb involvement (Bleck 1975). The degree, distribution, and patterns of abnormal tone result in the client's inability to move and/or assume and hold unsupported sitting postures sufficient to perform within acceptable age-appropriate functional limits.

Although by definition cerebral palsy is nonprogressive, the resulting clinical symptoms, if untreated, may result in physical and functional deterioration. For example, untreated, persistent, high asymmetrical tone often results in progressive orthopedic deformities. It is assumed that the clients being evaluated by the seating team are considered nonfunctional ambulators, at least at present.

Prognosis

Cerebral palsy is nonprogressive, but the clinical manifestations may worsen, especially if there is no intervention.

Life expectancy is normal; however, those with severe involvement have reduced respiratory function (Nwaobi and Smith 1986).

Intelligence
- severely retarded to above normal

Medical Concerns
- pathological reflexes result in patterns of abnormal tone
- potential for severe orthopedic complications
- incontinence of bowel and bladder function when training is not possible or the environment is not supportive
- decreased respiratory function in some
- sensory status is intact but there is concern for those with severe involvement who do not have the ability to move independently

ADL Status
- depends on the severity of the disability

Upper Extremity Function
- depends on the severity of the disability

Seating Considerations

Goals of Seating
· ·
- **Maximize function.** With appropriate seating, the client can have maximum use of the extremities in order to perform functional activities. Dynamic yet comfortable positions will assist in lengthening attention span on tasks other than balance; this, in turn, allows for cognitive development.

- **Improve self-image.** A well-seated individual will present as more comfortable and alert. Not only will such clients feel better about themselves but others will approach them with fewer preconceived notions about cognitive level.

- **Improve physiological function.** Increased respiratory function is the result of adapted seating (Nwaobi and Smith 1986).

Objectives of Seating
· ·
- **Reduce the influence of abnormal pathology.** Clients with cerebral palsy often have evidence of one or more pathological reflexes (Fiorentino 1973). If left unattended, they will result in asymmetrical or symmetrical fixed postures which in turn will often result in orthopedic deformities.

  Clients should be positioned in such a way as to diminish the effects of the abnormal pathology. The results over time will be a lessening of the effects of the abnormal posturing as well as the client's ability to have more control over the body and how it moves.

- **Normalize tone.** Persistent abnormal pathology results in postural tone being either too high, too low, or a combination of the two. Asymmetrical patterns of tone result in rotational deformities and unstable, asymmetrical postures. By reducing or eliminating the influence of abnormal pathology and positioning either to decrease tone or to support for lack of tone, the client will be able to sit in a more stable, symmetrical posture.

- **Prevent, delay, or accommodate deformity.** Deformity is the result of long-term posturing and lack of movement. It stands to reason that, if children are positioned in midline postures at an early age, the degree of deformity will be lessened. In the case of some clients with athetoid cerebral palsy, it is felt that midline seating can actually prevent the development of deformity by diminishing the effect of the asymmetrical posturing resulting from the asymmetric tonic neck reflex.

  In cases where deformities are already present, the seating system can help slow the progression of the deformity or, in severe cases, at least accommodate and support the deformity.

- **Increase comfort.** By providing adequate weight distribution and appropriately designed seat-back surfaces, the seating system can increase sitting tolerance.

- **Ensure skin integrity.** Although the sensation in persons with cerebral palsy is normal, the lack of ability to move and the need for supports to be placed on non-weight-bearing surfaces requires that attention be given to skin integrity, especially with clients who are thin and bony, and clients with more severe impairments.

- **Enhance quality of life.** In addition to the client having an improved self image, family members are more likely to include the person with the disability on community outings if management, including transportation, is relatively easy.

Evaluation for Seating and Mobility

Neuromotor Evaluation

The neuromotor evaluation focuses on pathological reflexes and muscle tone. This is not intended to be a comprehensive analysis of status but merely a screening tool to determine the effects of reflexes and tone on the seated position. This screening also attempts to answer the question of whether a seating system would be useful in reducing the effects of the pathological reflexes.

The pathological reflexes that dominate the individual's posture and movements are identified. The focus is on tonal changes and asymmetries which cause posture abnormalities in seating, particularly when the individual attempts a functional skill. It is only by directly inhibiting the effects of abnormal pathology that an optimal seated position can be obtained and maintained.

It is also necessary to consider how pathological reflexes influence tone. For example, it must be determined if the observed extensor tone is the result of a tonic labyrinthine supine reflex or if it is the predominance of extensor tone. In addition, changes in tone during attempts at functional skills, such as attempted speech or operating a piece of equipment, are noted (figure 5.1).

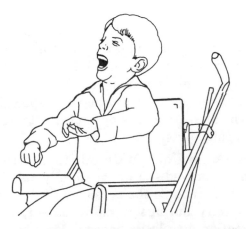

Figure 5.1. Client showing high tone on vocalization.

Tonal problems are indicated by the presence of spasticity, athetosis, and/or ataxia. Hypertonicity can be exhibited as either an overall dominance of extensor or flexor tone. Conversely, hypotonicity is observed as generalized floppiness. A combination of hypotonicity and hypertonicity is also seen frequently in persons with cerebral palsy.

Individuals with a diagnosis of spastic quadriplegic cerebral palsy present with mixed tone, usually a hypotonic trunk with hypertonic extremities. Individuals with athetosis are noted to have wide fluctuations of tone and can be hypotonic one moment and hypertonic the next (figures 5.2, 5.3).

Individuals affected by ataxia are observed to have decreased coordination, which worsens with attempts at functional tasks. Each client will have a unique distribution of tone, but there are predictable patterns which can assist the team when setting seating goals. Observe the tone the client exhibits in the arms of the caregiver, in the present seating system, and/or lying on a flat surface. Also observe any pathological reflexes which will influence the individual's ability to assume a seated position.

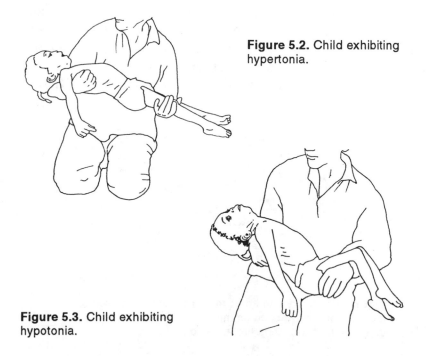

Figure 5.2. Child exhibiting hypertonia.

Figure 5.3. Child exhibiting hypotonia.

Handle the child and feel the tone/reflex patterns so as to begin to sense what triggers the abnormal movements and what assists in normalizing them. There are certain reflexes which are generally assessed in connection with seating concerns. These include the asymmetric tonic neck reflex (ATNR), the symmetric tonic neck reflex (STNR), the tonic labyrinthine reflex/supine (TLRS) and prone (TLRP), the positive supporting reflex, the extensor thrust reaction, and the crossed extension reflex.

Asymmetric Tonic Neck Reflex

The ATNR is elicited with lateral rotation of the head (figure 5.4). With this head movement, extension predominates on the facial side of the body, with flexion predominating on the skull side. There is lateral pelvic obliquity of the pelvis (down on the skull side) with lateral flexion of the trunk, convex to the skull side.

If left to dominate posturing, the ATNR can lead to asymmetrical sitting and lying postures which can result in scoliosis and wind-swept deformity. In clients with spasticity, the ATNR tends to be stronger to one side, and the side of preference never changes. In clients with athetosis, the side of preference can change with the position of the head. Therefore, clients with spasticity are much more likely to remain in one posture and develop orthopedic problems than are those with athetosis who are constantly changing position.

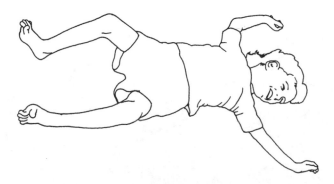

Figure 5.4. Child with an asymmetric tonic neck reflex to the left: the arm and leg on the face side are in extension; on the skull side, limbs are in flexion.

Some clients use the ATNR to place the extended arm in position to perform functional activities. This can reinforce the scoliosis and should be examined carefully in light of the long-term effects of the posturing. Considerations for seating should include providing a midline posture of the head.

Symmetric Tonic Neck Reflex

STNR is elicited by flexion or extension of the neck. When the neck is flexed, the upper extremities flex and there is extension of the lower extremities. The pelvis assumes a posterior pelvic tilt and the trunk is in a kyphotic posture (figure 5.5).

When the head is extended, the upper extremities extend and the lower extremities flex (figure 5.6). One would expect to see the pelvis in an anterior pelvic tilt with the trunk assuming a lordotic posture, but this is not often the case. Even when the client looks up, the pelvis most often remains in a posterior tilt and the trunk in a kyphotic posture. However, tone changes do occur in the extremities as the client looks up and down.

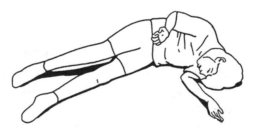

Figure 5.5. Symmetric tonic neck reflex: when the neck is flexed, there is extension of the lower extremities and flexion of the upper extremities.

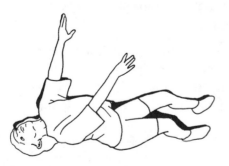

Figure 5.6. Symmetric tonic neck reflex: when the neck is extended, there is flexion of the lower extremities and extension of the upper extremities.

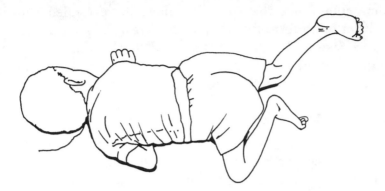

Figure 5.7. Child exhibiting a tonic labyrinthine prone reflex.

Considerations for seating should include the provision of a position for the head in space such that the client's visual field is in the neutral position. Work can be placed on an easel to angle it so the client does not have to look down.

Tonic Labyrinthine Reflex/Supine (TLRS) and Prone (TLRP)

The TLRS and TLRP (primarily) affect the individual's tone as a result of the angle of the head in space. (The labyrinths are part of the inner ear and help to maintain the head in a horizontal position.) In sitting, this reflex is elicited when the head is allowed to move posterior to the 90-degree upright position; extensor tone dominates throughout the body. Clients experience extension in all extremities and in the trunk, and they are often seen sliding out of the seat.

Conversely, when the head moves anterior to the 90-degree upright position, overall flexor tone dominates: the extremities flex and the trunk becomes kyphotic.

Considerations for seating should include positioning the head in space in as neutral a position as possible so that neither flexor nor extensor tone dominates. If the child's trunk needs to be reclined, an effort should be made to bring the head into a neutral position.

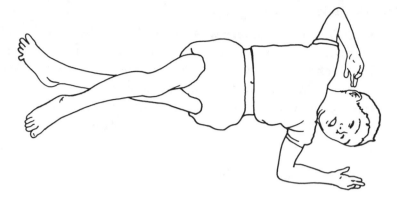

Figure 5.8. Child exhibiting a tonic labyrinthine supine reflex.

Positive Supporting Reflex and Extensor Thrust Reaction

The positive supporting reflex and extensor thrust reaction relate to positioning of the feet. Pressure on the ball of the foot causes either a lower extremity extensor pattern, a full extension pattern, or an extensor thrust in which the individual appears to be forcefully ejected from the seat or from standing on the foot platform (figure 5.9).

Considerations for seating should include placing the feet carefully on footrests. If the reaction continues, dorsiflex the foot slightly; in extreme cases, do without the footrest for a time. In persistent cases, a referral to an orthotist may be appropriate.

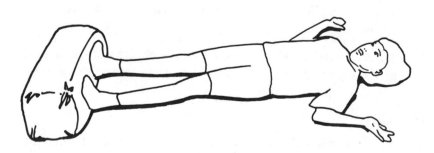

Figure 5.9. Extension of the lower extremities with pressure under the ball of the foot.

Rooting Reflex

The rooting reaction occurs when stimulus to the cheek near the mouth area elicits turning of the head toward the stimulus and opening of the mouth. The presence of this reflex results in involuntary head posturing and, in extreme cases, will contribute to scoliosis. Considerations for seating should include selecting headrests and neck rests that do not come in contact with the cheek.

Medical/Orthopedic Evaluation
. . . .

Medical issues of concern to the seating clinical team address a very narrow spectrum of the overall medical care of the client. It is not the desire nor the intent of the seating team to take over the medical management of the client. Rather, the seating team strives to guide its decision-making to complement the existing plan. Based on the seating team's evaluation, however, recommendations for surgical intervention may be forthcoming.

Management of the client with orthopedic deformities is a combination of surgical intervention (when indicated and possible) and seating. It will become obvious that a combination of approaches is often appropriate.

It is also acknowledged that in some geographic areas and for clients with more severe or multiple disabilities, surgical intervention is not an option for a variety of reasons. The unavailability of such services, however, does not preclude the necessity for seating. It would warrant very realistic goal-setting by the seating team with clear communication to the client and the family.

In evaluating orthopedic status, the therapist determines if the goal is to try to prevent deformity, correct deforming postures, or accommodate deformity.

Pelvis

Fixed deformities of the pelvis are among the most difficult problems to overcome in achieving a satisfactory sitting posture. These deformities include pelvic rotation, pelvic tilt, and pelvic obliquity. These deformities may occur separately or in conjunction with one another. See Appendix A, Standardization of Terminology, for a further definition of this.

Rotational deformities of the pelvis are secondary to abnormalities in either lower limbs or the spine and, accordingly, may be envisioned as due to intrapelvic forces, suprapelvic forces, or to a combination of the two.

Severe adduction deformities of the hip often cause pelvic rotation. When this pelvic deformity becomes fixed, it cannot be corrected even though the deforming force at the hip is relieved. Therefore, it must be accommodated by altering the seating system. Pelvic obliquity is usually secondary to a scoliotic spinal curve which extends to the sacrum.

Once such deformities become fixed, the pelvic tilt requires accommodation in the seating system by inserting a lift beneath the high side of the pelvis. It is frequently impossible to achieve good sitting posture in these individuals, and one must accept a compromise of partial improvement in order to place the head in or near the midline. Posterior pelvic tilt may be part of a long lumbar-dorsal spinal kyphosis which produces pelvic flexion, or it may develop secondary to sacral sitting because of persistently high extensor tone or hip flexion contractures.

In contrast, pelvic flexion deformities develop when the individual lacks extension, as seen in severe fixed lumbar lordosis. Again, compromise modification of the seating system to accommodate these deformities is the best approach.

Spine

Spinal deformities develop in individuals with neuromuscular disorders because of unequal forces—generated by an imbalance in strength or tone—acting on opposite sides of the spinal column. Response to infrapelvic forces may also cause or contribute to the development of abnormal spinal curves. Spinal deformities present as a scoliosis, kyphosis, lordosis, or some combination of these curves.

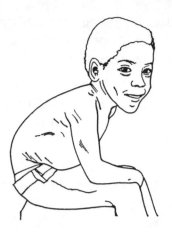

Figure 5.10. A child with a flexible kyphosis.

Of all the problems confronted in the seating clinic, spinal deformities are likely to be one of the most challenging and difficult to solve satisfactorily. Often, once deformities have begun, they cannot truly be controlled by any seating system now available. It has been found that progression of these deformities can be slowed but not stopped by seating systems even when instituted at a very early age.

UTREP experience has shown, however, that very early symmetrical seating for clients with athetosis can prevent spinal curvatures. Various spinal support systems have been used, depending upon the type and severity of the curve, with varying success. Often, one must simply accommodate the curve by custom modifications. Molded plastic body jackets or other spinal orthoses are often an adjunct to seating systems in the management of these deformities.

Furthermore, parental or institutional resistance to surgical intervention may preclude surgery entirely or delay it until opportunity for achieving a satisfactory result has passed.

Upper Extremities

Many clients who require specialized seating systems have limited or no use of their hands. However, there are individuals who have the potential for both volitional hand placement and at least gross motor function of the hand for operating switches if undesirable reflexes and excessive

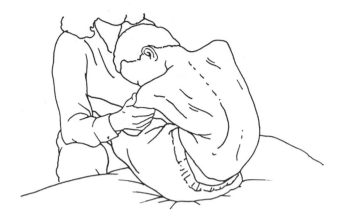

Figure 5.11. A client with a scoliosis which is only partially flexible.

motor tone can be reduced. Therefore, the assessment should include a range-of-motion screening as well as gross and fine motor skills assessment, with particular considerations given to the client's ability to use the hands/arms for switch and/or joystick operation.

There is rarely an indication for surgical intervention for upper limb deformities in these clients, although selected soft tissue releases may occasionally be appropriate.

Lower Extremities

With few exceptions, clients who require special seating systems are nonambulatory, and most are unable to stand except with maximum support. Gross deformities, fixed joint contractures, and significant limb length inequalities are immediately apparent and will usually necessitate customization of the seating system.

Hip and thigh. Flexion contractures, unless unusually severe, are not a common problem since individuals with spasticity are usually positioned at 90 degrees or greater of hip flexion. Individuals who lack hip flexion may be completely precluded from sitting because there is no weight-bearing surface available. A mild to moderate loss of normal hip flexion range may result in "sacral sitting."

Abduction contractures are not common, but when present and severe, they prevent acceptable seating primarily due to overall width at the knees requiring a wider-than-normal chair based on the width at the hips.

In comparison, adduction contractures are common and may lead to or be associated with paralytic dislocation of the hip. Prior to producing complete hip dislocation, adduction deformities may necessitate seating modifications to counteract the adduction force or may require fairly simple surgical procedures.

Once complete hip dislocation has occurred, it becomes difficult or impossible to bring the involved hip to the neutral position; the individual often presents with a wind-swept deformity where the dislocated hip is severely adducted and the opposite hip is abducted (figure 5.12).

Such wind-swept deformities are usually accompanied by a secondary pelvic rotation. The pelvic rotation can be magnified if the wind-swept deformity is not accommodated. Attempts to bring the lower extremities into a more neutral position can result in further rotation of the pelvis and perhaps the trunk. Dislocated hips do not usually cause pain in people with cerebral palsy who are not ambulatory. If pain does occur with sufficient intensity, it may be necessary to recommend surgical correction of the dislocation.

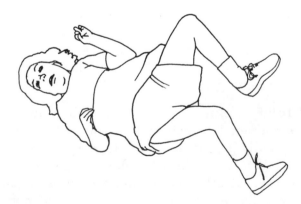

Figure 5.12. A client with a wind-swept deformity.

As with other skeletal deformities which develop because of a dynamic neuromuscular imbalance, experience indicates that the development of hip dislocation or pelvic rotation deformities cannot be prevented by appropriate seating alone. But when incorporated into a well-designed total treatment program, proper seating can assuredly play a major role in slowing the development of these deformities. Excessive internal or external rotation contractures at the hip may cause difficulties in achieving satisfactory seating, but most can be accommodated by fairly simple seat modifications.

Major thigh length inequality resulting from hip dislocation necessitates a step-off modification of the seat section to adequately accommodate the deformity (figure 5.13).

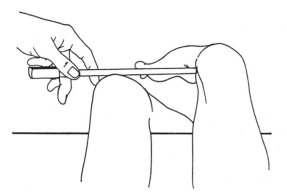

Figure 5.13. Child with leg length discrepancy due to a dislocated hip on the left.

Knee and leg. Tibial torsion is rarely severe enough to require any treatment other than modification of the foot support section of the seating system to accommodate the deformity. Tibial leg length inequality is easily equalized by increasing the thickness of the foot support beneath the short leg. Although in most seating systems the knee is placed in 90 degrees of flexion or more, extension contractures or a lack of full extension of the knee rarely present a problem in seating.

In contrast, knee flexion contractures may necessitate significant modification of the seating system. If this is not accommodated, the forces pushing the knee into extension will also pull the pelvis posteriorly, encouraging sacral sitting because the hamstrings cross both the hip and knee joints.

Tightness of the rectus femoris muscles (hamstrings) creates a special problem for the seating team because this muscle group travels over two joints. Position change at the pelvis directly affects the position of the leg. If the individual is allowed to sit in a posterior pelvic tilt, a kyphosis will result. If the individual is seated in a more neutral pelvic tilt, often the hamstrings force the knee into increased flexion, creating a seating challenge of how to provide a foot platform.

Foot and ankle. Varus, valgus, and equinous deformities are frequently encountered.

When fixed and severe, such deformities necessitate either the use of a foot support modified to accommodate the deformity or correction of the deformity by casting, bracing, or surgical release of contracted soft tissue.

In summary, when evaluating an individual's orthopedic deformities, it must be determined if, and to what degree, they can realistically be corrected or if in fact accommodation and maintenance should be the goal.

Functional Skills Evaluation

The functional skills evaluation focuses on the investigation of the client's present abilities in relation to the tasks to be performed. Seating should enhance a person's ability to be independent in activities of daily living such as mobility, feeding, self-care and hygiene, and written and spoken communication.

Functional independence should be considered as part of the overall provision of a seating system. There are times when there must be compromise between the ideal posture and the posture that enables a person to be functional, but whenever possible, technology should be used to encourage motor skill performance in as normal a pattern of motion and tone as possible.

For example, a person cannot be prevented from performing a functional task because abnormal pathology is used, without offering another mode of performing that task. If a person propels a wheelchair backwards with his feet and rotates his body so that he can see where he is going, he cannot be placed in a forward sitting posture and have his ability to be independently mobile taken away. He can, however, be provided with a powered wheelchair which can be driven in a forward sitting midline posture. A child who uses her ATNR to position her hand should not be discouraged from doing so if it is the only means she has of accomplishing this task. Of course, other patterns of motion should be investigated if at all possible, and the long-term effects should be considered in the overall management of the child's posture.

Functional skills which are screened include mobility, feeding, communication (written and spoken), computer access, personal hygiene, and alternate positioners for night-time uses. Environmental accessibility is always important, especially when considering the type of mobility device.

Mobility

There are three categories of wheelbases from which to choose as a person's mode of mobility:
- manual dependent
- manual independent
- power

If a client is able to propel a manual base at a functional speed with reasonable energy costs, then a manually propelled base should be the one of choice. If energy costs are too high and if motor skills are insufficient, then powered mobility should be considered. Of course, there are many issues which must be considered before powered chairs are prescribed, including environmental barriers, cognitive and perceptual skills, transportation, and cost. Guidelines as to the evaluation of mobility are covered in the section on Powered Mobility (pages 31-40).

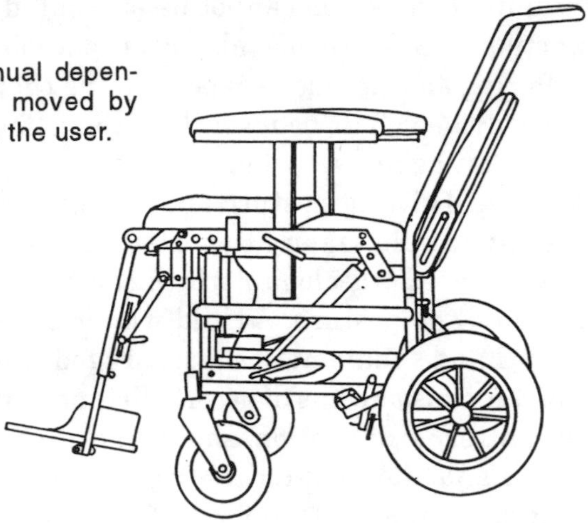

Figure 5.14. A manual dependent wheelchair is moved by someone other than the user.

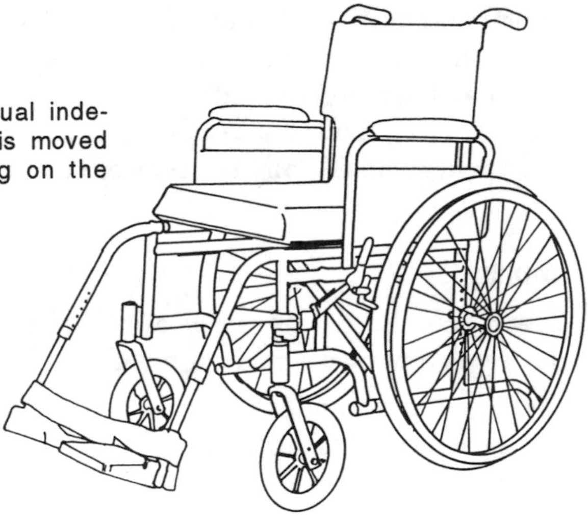

Figure 5.15. A manual independent wheelchair is moved by the user pushing on the wheels.

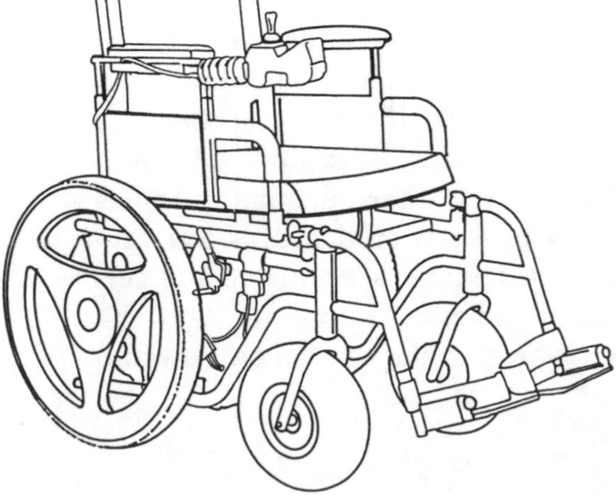

Figure 5.16. A powered wheelchair is moved by the user directing a joystick or other type of control.

Optimally, only those persons who have insufficient motor ability or cognitive or perceptual skills to be independently mobile should have a manual dependent base prescribed. Manual dependent bases can also be considered for special purposes (such as in an airplane).

Eating

When one is sitting in a well-supported posture in a therapeutic seating system, with the tray or table at the appropriate height, the increase in hand skill can sometimes enable a person to eat independently. If motor skills are insufficient to manage independent eating, a well-positioned individual is much easier to feed because of more normal tone in the oral musculature.

There are a number of adaptive feeding devices on the market which can assist a person to become independent. A word of caution is necessary, however. Mealtime is a very social time of one's day. Persons with disabilities sometimes prefer to be fed by an experienced feeder than to struggle with being independent using a technical aid in front of others. A training period in private is recommended and, as with all technical aids, the user's preference should be respected.

If an eating device is used, careful attention must be given to the type and position of tray being recommended as well as the height and accessibility of table tops.

Communication

Augmentative communication technology, if required, can be purchased from a variety of sources. Complete listings of available technology are available (Brandenburg and Vanderheiden 1987) as well as guidelines for evaluation and implementation strategies (Blackstone 1986; Blackstone, Cassatt-James, and Brusken 1988).

When evaluating a client for a seating system, the therapist must consider the type of augmentative communication system a person will be receiving and how it will be operated. The position in which the augmentative aid is mounted, vocabulary placement, the hardware used for mounting it, and the position of the control switch are factors to be considered. To minimize later complex and expensive modifications, the speech pathologist should be involved at the time the seating and mobility systems are being recommended.

Computer Access

Positioning makes a major contribution to a person's ability to operate a computer. A stable trunk position frees the hands for function and sometimes can make the difference between a person directly operating the keyboard or needing adaptive hardware. The use of keyguards can assist persons with ataxia or athetosis who have difficulty hitting only one key, as well as spastic individuals who tend to have difficulty separating individual finger motion and rest their palms on the keys. Even for individuals who have greater motor impairment and who must use single switches or expanded keyboards to operate a computer, the seated position will make a difference in accuracy and efficiency. Particular attention must be paid to the height of the seating in relationship to the workstation height (figure 5.17).

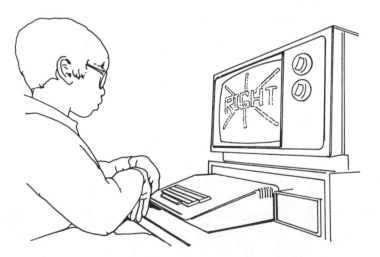

Figure 5.17. A stable upright posture enables a child to use a computer keyboard.

Personal Hygiene

As with most technical aids, there are a number of options for toileting and bathing. While not directly connected to seating, these devices should be considered as part of the overall technical aid provision.

The seat height of a seating system must be carefully evaluated if the individual will be transferring to a toilet or bath chair. Seat design should also allow for use of a urinal if it is a usable device. Toilet seats which offer very stable sitting with a firm attachment are recommended, as are bath aids which do not slip and which are designed so the caregiver can easily access the device. These devices should be tried in a real-life situation whenever possible before purchase.

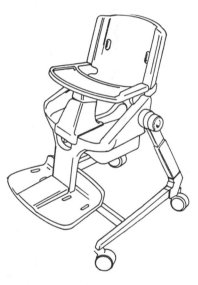

Figure 5.18. A specially designed toilet aid for children with physical disabilities (PinDot Products).

Alternate Positioners

A variety of alternate positions should be available to persons with physical disabilities. Therapeutic positioning equipment provides a means by which therapeutic goals can be extended well beyond the treatment time. Sitting is only one position. There are positioning aids for standing in upright and prone postures, lying on the side, prone, and supine positions, sitting devices for cars, desks, and unique purposes such as horseback riding. Of increasing interest are methods and technologies for positioning persons in bed. However, few items are presently commercially available to meet this need.

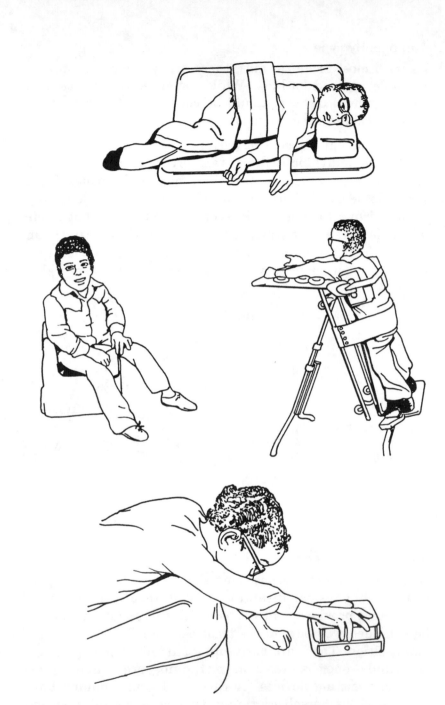

Figure 5.19. Children should be positioned in a variety of postures throughout the day. Alternate positioning devices: side lyer (top), corner seat (left), prone stander (right), and prone positioner (bottom).

Decision-Making Guidelines

Once a thorough evaluation has been completed, the therapist outlines the goals of positioning in sitting. Once the goals are thoroughly understood, the team must come to an agreement as to the most appropriate type of technology to use to meet the client's seating and functional needs. This section will address the therapeutic considerations relating to each component of the seating system. A problem-solving chart can be used as a guide for troubleshooting when a seating device is not meeting its intended purpose (see Appendix C, pages 295-300).

Positioning the Individual Pelvis

In almost all situations, decision-making for the seated position begins at the pelvis. The pelvis provides the base of support from which the rest of the body segments follow.

Whenever possible, the pelvis should be positioned in midline on a firm support. Persons with neuromotor dysfunctions are more functional on a firm base of support because it facilitates proximal stability, and small weight shifts contribute to increased trunk and upper extremity function. Sitting tolerance is increased as well. Firm does not mean hard, and tolerance does not mean stoic perseverance. The firm seat is one which is comfortably tolerated for hours at a time. A number of cushions have been designed for individuals with insensitive tissue but can be used effectively for those with neuromotor disabilities who lack the ability to move away from discomfort.

In situations where the ischial tuberosities are not level and fixed in this position, then the contoured approach is used with an appropriate buildup under the higher side to maintain even weight distribution. If the asymmetry of the pelvis is flexible, attempts should be made to level the pelvis by building up the seat on the lower side. The pelvis should be blocked from lateral motion by lateral bolsters which can be either part of the design of the seating component or pelvic blocks which are part of the wheelbase. If the pelvis is allowed to drift laterally, the trunk will take on a scoliotic posture.

In most cases an anatomical hip angle of 90 degrees is effective in normalizing extensor tone. Anterior rolls, wedges, and antithrust or ramped designs can position the hips at 90 degrees and facilitate the reduction of extensor tone, inhibiting posterior pelvic rotation and subsequent kyphotic posturing.

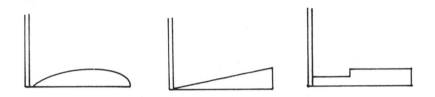

Figure 5.20. Three possible designs for seat components: roll (left); wedge (middle); antithrust (right).

These designs are quite different from a flexed seat which does not consider the contour of the buttocks and often leads to a posterior pelvic rotation.

Occasionally, lumbar supports are used to maintain the pelvis in an anterior or neutral tilt. Remember, however, that lumbar curve does not develop in the normal child until about eight or nine years of age (Zacharkow 1988). Hypotonic individuals appear to benefit from this contour. More often, a sacral pad is used (Mulchahy and Pountney 1986). Sacral pads are designed to hold the pelvis in a neutral position. They usually extend from the top of the seat to just below the PSIS.

Many individuals with increased lower extremity tone have difficulty obtaining and maintaining this posture due to tight hamstrings. If too much anterior tilt is enforced, then it is likely that the hamstrings will tighten even more, causing increased knee flexion. Compromise may be required.

Lap belts are part of the technology used to keep the pelvis in position. Most often a lap belt is positioned at about a 60-degree angle to the pelvis under the anterior superior iliac spine, with direct contact about the pelvis (figure 5.21a). If the client exhibits a great deal of extensor tone, a more rigid design of a belt may be used. For those with a fixed posterior pelvic tilt, a lap belt mounted perpendicular to the seat is often effective (figure 5.21b).

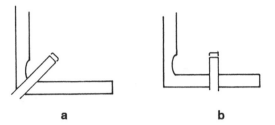

Figure 5.21. Lap-belt placement is critical to secure the pelvis.

The use of groin straps to hold the pelvis in position is discouraged due to discomfort, hygiene concerns, and unacceptable cosmesis. Most often, properly adjusted lap belts in conjunction with appropriate hip angle and angle in space will maintain the clients in their seating systems.

Another option utilized to secure the pelvis in a neutral position is a knee block (Monahan, Taylor, and Shaw 1989; Mulchahy and Pountney 1986). The knee block has been quite effective in decreasing pelvic rotation to the right or left and preventing posterior pelvic tilt.

Lower Extremities

Medial thigh bolsters (pommels or abductor wedges) are used to provide lower extremity abduction. In conjunction with a 90-degree or greater hip flexion angle, medial thigh bolsters serve to inhibit extensor tone. They are also necessary when the lower extremities are tending toward a wind-swept or an adducted posture, as they encourage neutral positioning. When medial bolsters are used, they should be positioned as distally as possible so as not to stimulate the hip adductors or crossed extension reflex.

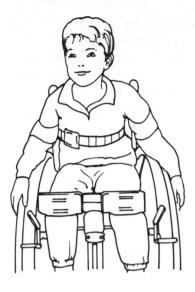

Figure 5.22. Knee blocks used in conjunction with a lap belt help with pelvic positioning.

In persons with hypertonic extremities, the degree of abduction given by the pommel should be carefully observed to ensure that it is encouraging relaxation. Flip-down or detachable pommels should be considered if the individual is independent or assisted in a forward or side transfer or if a urinal is used while the individual is seated. Medial thigh bolsters should never be used instead of a lap belt to hold a person in the seating system.

Wherever possible, the foot supports of the wheelchair should be used because they are stronger than most foot platforms. Often it is necessary to modify these wheelchair footrests to achieve the desired lower extremity positioning. Individual foot supports with either ankle straps or toe loops are simple ways to position the foot in a neutral plantigrade position. If there is increased extensor tone in the lower extremities when the feet are placed on the foot platform, slight dorsiflexion of the ankle can help normalize the tone. Custom foot platforms can accommodate severely deformed feet or can be mounted slightly under the seat to accommodate clients with tight hamstrings. Feet should always be supported not only to prevent deformity but to maintain the appropriate hip, knee, and ankle positions. Based on the evaluation, decisions applicable to the functional design criteria should follow.

....

Optimally, the trunk should be positioned in a midline, upright posture. As mentioned in the evaluation section on the abnormal pathological reflexes, the position of the head in space is critical to tone management. Research studies have verified that clients experienced less abnormal tone with a resultant increase in upper extremity function if they were seated in the upright posture (Nwaobi 1987).

However, not all clients can tolerate this position. Individuals with hypotonic or weak trunks, poor or no head control, and/or severe orthopedic involvement of the trunk will need to be tilted in space. The hip angle is maintained and the total system is tilted. Then the head can be brought forward to minimize the effects of gravity.

A scoliotic or kyphotic posture is more comfortably accommodated when some of the effects of gravity are eliminated by tilting. It is useful to use a simulator for deciding on the angle of tilt because very small increments can be tried. It is possible that a base with a tilt feature could be used if a client needs to be tilted for only part of the day. Be cautious of tilted seated postures. To the uninformed, the clients look more comfortable when tilted 20 to 30 degrees. They do not see the increase in extensor tone and the passivity often created when clients are unable to come upright for work.

People with hydrocephalus usually have low-tone trunks with weak neck musculature and cannot support the weight of their larger-than-normal heads pushing down on their trunks over time. Sometimes orthotic body jackets are prescribed to support a hypotonic trunk until the growing years are completed or until surgical stabilization can become an option. Lateral support should be only as aggressive as necessary. Some clients need only a reminder of midline. Others need aggressive midline support in order to feel secure enough to operate a powered wheelchair or other technical device. Some require thoracic supports to be offset in a three-point pressure system to support a developing scoliosis (see figure 21 in Biomechanics, page 62).

In this situation, the three points consist of the pelvis on the side opposite the curve, a support under the apex of the curve, and the final support high on the opposite side of the curve. To ensure repeatable positioning, both sides of the pelvis are usually blocked.

Over-support of the trunk can cause a decrease in function over time. Decisions as to appropriate anterior chest support are made in conjunction with the design of the back component. One can choose from both rigid anterior shoulder restraints and more flexible designs of chest belts, H-harnesses, and chest panels. Again, as minimal support as possible should be used. Even individuals who have fair to good trunk control require additional support for functional skills, such as operating a powered mobility device or feeding themselves.

Chest panels or H-harnesses also seem to be effective in reducing neck and trunk hypertonicity in individuals with head injuries, by exerting firm pressure over the shoulders.

Note: Whenever using an anterior belt or panel, do not use buckles that can slip out of adjustment. They can create a safety concern with clients who move at all in their seating systems.

Some clients cannot tolerate anterior chest supports such as chest panels which attempt to pull them posteriorly. For these individuals, anterior supports attached to a tray that they can lean into are recommended.

Finally, anterior chest supports can assist with stability during transportation although it should be remembered that only crash-tested restraints provide collision protection.

Upper Extremities and Shoulders

Frequently, little is said about positioning of the upper extremities, yet when one considers that the hands are the body's part of choice for operation of most technical aids, even for those with severe physical disabilities, then upper extremity placement becomes a critical issue.

Many clients will have trays as part of their seating systems. The most common height for mounting would be one in which the forearms rest comfortably on a tray surface with the elbows at a 90-degree angle when the shoulders are relaxed. If a communication aid is being used on the tray, there might be a reason to lower the tray.

Persons with athetosis work better in extremes of range, usually in extension, and therefore would be more functional if their elbows were extended. On the other hand, some clients with spasticity who are very tight into flexion would work better if the tray were mounted a little higher than normal to assist in relaxing upper extremity tone.

Trays that restrain the nonfunctional arms of clients have been successful as an adjunct to the seating system. In particular, arm restraint trays work well for persons with athetosis who use their heads for operation of technical aids and need the added trunk stability as well as the reassurance that their arms will not be in the way.

Arm restraint trays also work well with individuals who display self-abusive behavior such as is the case in individuals with Lesch-Nyan syndrome.

Many adults do not like to use large trays. Small, specific-purpose armrests or fold-away trays are possible options. Trays should be used to achieve specific goals, not simply installed routinely on all systems. Trays may have negative psychosocial considerations as they do not allow the individual to get close to people or objects or allow other people to get close to them. A tray can serve as a barrier to interpersonal interaction in some cases.

Occasionally, protraction of the shoulders is necessary to assist relaxation of extensor tone. This can be accomplished through the addition of protraction wings on the tray or the back of the system. Clients observed to elevate shoulders (usually in an attempt to stabilize) can be assisted with chest panel straps which directly contact the shoulders, providing a downward pull.

Decisions regarding the support of the head can be most challenging. As mentioned before, the position of the head in space can dictate the presence and degree of abnormal tone. Only with someone who has a strong persistent ATNR or extensor tone caused by a TLRS should head position be addressed first. Neck collars or occipital rings can be effective for clients who require only a reminder of midline or slight forward flexion of the head to reduce extensor tone. The placement of the collar just below the external occipital protuberance does not provide sensory stimulus to the back of the head, which can sometimes stimulate extensor tone.

Clients demonstrating a TLRS or TLRP must have a careful evaluation of head position. Often, these clients require a head position as close to upright as possible. Those who must be reclined for trunk control can have support which brings the head closer to upright. The two-step headrest works best for clients who either demonstrate hyperextension of the neck or who have no head control. The two-step headrest is a combination of the occipital collar and the headrest: it follows the contour of the head and provides a shelf on which the occipital bone rests.

For more challenging clients, custom headrests can be fabricated. Anterior hardware or straps about the head are used only when absolutely necessary, because of both safety concerns and cosmetic considerations.

In clients observed to pull forward into flexion or flop forward, an anterior support can eliminate the head-hanging position. Neck collars such as the Hensinger head supports (Danmar Products, Inc., 221 Jackson Industrial Dr., Ann Arbor, MI 48103) or Miller Total head support (Miller Special Products, 284 East Market St., Akron, OH 44301) are useful for those who hyperextend out of anterior support or who demonstrate a lateral head flexion posture. The use of the headrest may be necessary for individuals with fair to good head control when increased functional demand is placed upon them, such as with the operation of powered wheelchairs.

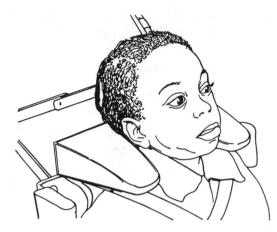

Figure 5.23. A neck collar placed below the occipital region of the head helps centralize the head.

Planar or Contoured?

The most common question at any workshop is about how to decide whether to use a planar or a contoured seating system. There are no set guidelines, although experienced clinicians usually have a rule of thumb. Choice often depends upon the experience of the therapist or person required to do the shaping of the contoured system and the availability of technical support.

Planar systems are sometimes less expensive and more adjustable. They require less technical expertise; they can be purchased from catalogs or local vendors, and several manufacturers will custom fabricate components. On the other hand, personnel doing contoured systems require some expertise in shaping and, for most systems, some technical support is required.

However, there are advantages to a *contoured system.* For persons with sensory impairments, the contour will more evenly distribute weight. It will more easily accommodate asymmetry which is the result of orthopedic deformity or abnormal tone. Contrary to the belief of some, contoured systems can be made so that they are adjustable in growth or can be easily and inexpensively modified, depending on the system. In fitting thousands of contoured systems over many years, it was found if growth was kept in mind during the contouring phase, systems could last for three to five years and longer if growth was in length and not width.

The decision should be made on an individual basis. Because of the severity of the clients seen at UTREP, at one point over 60% of the clients were fitted in custom contoured seating systems. If a planar system meets the need of the client, then it is often the system of choice. If there are sensory deficits or asymmetry, then a contoured system should at least be considered and the technical support required sought from the vendor or manufacturer if necessary. In every clinic, it is likely that both types of systems would need to be available in order to best meet clients' needs.

References

Blackstone, S. W., ed. 1986. *Augmentative communication: An introduction.* Rockville, MD: American Speech-Language-Hearing Association.

Blackstone, S. W., E. L. Cassatt-James, and D. M. Brusken. 1988. *Augmentative communication: Implementation strategies.* Rockville, MD: American Speech-Language-Hearing Association.

Bleck, E. E. 1975. Locomotor prognosis in cerebral palsy. *Developmental Medicine and Child Neurology* 17:18-25.

Brandenburg, S. A., and G. G. Vanderheiden. 1987. *Communication, control, and computer access for disabled and elderly individuals.* Boston, MA: College Hill/Little-Brown.

Fiorentino, M. 1973. *Reflex testing methods for evaluating central nervous system development.* Springfield, IL: Charles C. Thomas.

Monahan, M. P. A., S. J. Taylor, and C. G. Shaw. 1989. Pelvic positioning: Another option. In *Proceedings of the fifth international seating symposium: "Seating the disabled,"* 32-38. Memphis, TN: University of Tennessee.

Mulchahy, C. M., and T. E. Pountney. 1986. The sacral pad—Description of its clinical use in seating. *Physiotherapy* 72(9):473-74.

Nwaobi, O. M. 1987. Extremity function in children with cerebral palsy. *Journal of the American Physical Therapy Association* 68(8):1209-12.

Nwaobi, O. M., and P. P. Smith. 1986. Effect of adaptive seating on pulmonary function of children with cerebral palsy. *Developmental Medicine and Child Neurology* 28:351-54.

Zacharkow, P. 1988. *Posture, sitting, standing. Chair design and exercise.* Springfield, IL: Charles C. Thomas.

Head Injuries

Head Injuries

Diagnosis

A closed-head injury can be defined as diffuse brain damage that results from forces to the head. Resultant brain damage can be due to compression, tension, or shearing of brain tissue. Because of the diffuse nature of the brain damage, the clinical manifestations are complex. Damage can occur in the brainstem or cerebral cortex, can result from traumatic injury to blood vessels, can be secondary to cerebral edema, or can result from damage to the cranial nerves.

Personnel in seating clinics have become aware of the rapidly growing population of persons with head injuries in their clinics. Emergence of acute trauma centers in addition to the advancement of medical and surgical techniques are responsible for the increased survival rate of persons who suffer severe closed-head injuries. National statistics reveal that, of a yearly total of 422,000 persons with head injuries, 90% will recover fully and 10%, or approximately 42,000, will be left with residual deficits.

Closed-head injuries (CHI) occur most frequently in adult males between 15 and 24 years of age (Rimel, Jane, and Bond 1983). The most common cause of head injury by far is automobile accidents, with males being involved twice as often as females. Traumatic injuries are most likely to occur during summer vacation times and in the late afternoon.

Most often the person enters a coma at the time of injury, although occasionally this is delayed. In occurrences of mild injury (70% to 80% of admissions to hospital), the patients never do become unconscious. In the more severe injuries, coma is considered stage one of recovery. In stage two, the person is semi-comatose and experiences the return of some reflex activity. In stage three the person enters a period of stupor with restlessness, irritability, and delirium, although the patient may respond to simple commands. In the fourth stage, the person experiences a quiet confusion and responds to some commands, but responses are neither always appropriate nor coordinated. In the final stage, the person is fully conscious and is in the process of recovering orientation.

It should be stressed that the stages described above are not well defined and that patients can frequently experience symptoms of more than one stage at a time. Also, progress through the stages does not always occur in a hierarchical fashion, and in some situations a person may stop short of passing through all stages to recovery. Because of the diffuse nature of the brain damage, it is possible to see incomplete recovery with residual signs of brain damage even years after the medical recovery is said to be complete.

Rate and degree of recovery have been linked to a number of factors. The shorter the length of the coma, the better the chances of recovery. Also, persons under the age of 20 but over approximately five years of age seem to recover to a greater degree. Finally, the more quickly the person is treated, the less chance there is for secondary complications such as edema.

Clients can be referred to a seating program at any time during the recovery phase, but staff in acute care and even rehabilitation facilities are likely to postpone referral, waiting for recovery to plateau. However, experience has shown that early positioning, even with temporary positioning devices, can slow or prevent the development of deformities.

Medical Considerations

A variety of medical factors combine to make the management of people with closed-head injuries extremely challenging. Recovery occurs over approximately a two-year period, but the speed and the nature of the recovery are unpredictable. Some people experience full recovery; some recover most of their physical abilities but retain many residual behavioral, perceptual, or cognitive deficits; and some recover very little. Especially in the early stages, there are extreme variations in performance from day to day and even hour to hour, making goal-setting rather difficult. Although there are characteristic motor patterns, they are not predictable in intensity of tone or pattern of movement.

During the acute stage of severe head injury, patients are often in a coma and exhibit a decorticate posture (predominantly flexed) (figure 6.1), a decerebrate posture (predominantly extended), or a combination of the two (figure 6.2). The trunk and extremities are dominated by increased tone.

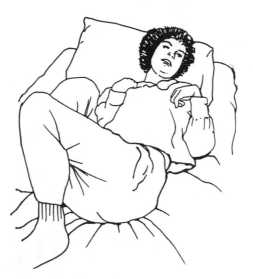

Figure 6.1. Client in a decorticate (flexed) position.

Some individuals with head injuries exhibit such extreme hypertonicity in the trunk that they assume an opisthotonos posture. Even if the tone of the trunk is relatively normal, there is often high tone in the extremities.

Those clients who maintain a decorticate posture for long periods of time are often left with severe flexion deformities, and those with the decerebrate posture have extension deformities. Furthermore, it is not unusual for clients to have a decerebrate posture on one side and a decorticate posture on the other (figure 6.3).

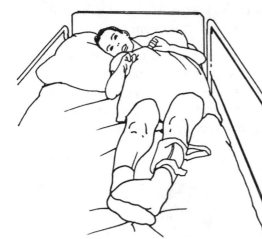

Figure 6.2. Client with decorticate posture in the arms and decerebrate posture in the legs.

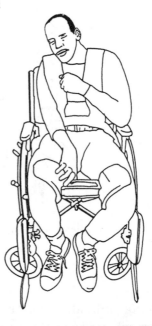

Figure 6.3. Poorly positioned client with decerebrate posture on the right and decorticate posture on the left.

The severity of persistent high tone, which makes positioning in the bed and wheelchair extremely difficult, can contribute to the development of orthopedic deformities. Clients who have low tone or no tone usually have few orthopedic problems. Because of the absence of predictable patterns of deformity, the management of tone varies with each person, and standard management principles as related to positioning have not been possible.

Spinal deformities were prevalent in a sample of clients with head injuries who were referred to UTREP for seating. (Referrals to this program represent only clients with severe tonal problems.) Over half of the clients had a fixed scoliosis while an additional 10% had evidence of a flexible scoliosis. One-third had flexible kyphosis and another one-third exhibited postural kyphosis. Pelvic deformity was minimal in people with head injuries, although tight hamstrings were encountered in almost half of the population. Flexion contractures in the elbows were more prevalent than lack of full flexion.

While preliminary analysis of anthropometric data on persons with cerebral palsy shows them to be smaller in stature than the population without physical disabilities (Hobson et al. 1991), those with head injuries are within range of standard anthropometric measurements. Therefore, individuals with head injuries are of normal stature, which means that they are significantly larger and heavier than the population with cerebral palsy.

A variety of other concerns are evident with this population. Especially in the early stages of recovery, the lack of stamina makes scheduling of intervention a challenge. Infections and other medical problems are often present which prolong the rehabilitation process.

A post-traumatic vision syndrome has been identified (Padula 1989) that includes diplopia, visual memory problems, poor tracking, staring, and the perception that objects are moving. Manifestations of this syndrome can influence the posturing of the head. What clients perceive as vertical is really offset from the vertical axis.

Heterotopic ossification is common in people with head injuries. Abnormal calcification occurs in and around the joints, causing pain on movement. This produces a reluctance to move, and the result is often the development of contractures about the joints. The calcification must be surgically removed once the calcification process stops.

Even when the medical condition is considered stable and at a level of premorbid function, the client is often left with residual deficits in cognition, emotion, and perception. These more subtle deficits can often be the limiting factor in reintegrating the person at home and in the work environment.

Goals of Seating

- **Normalize tone.** In most cases, this will mean reducing the abnormally high flexor or extensor tone. There are few set patterns of abnormal tone, so each person must be assessed individually to determine the most appropriate position to inhibit the hypertonicity.

- **Prevent, support, or accommodate deformity.** In the early stages of recovery, the goal is to position the person in bed and, if possible, in a chair to prevent the formation of deformities. Over time, and often very rapidly, postural deformities will become fixed. Then the goal of seating must become one of support and accommodation.

- **Prevent pressure sore formation.** Both while in bed and in a wheelchair, care must be taken to prevent the formation of pressure sores. About 10% of persons with CHI who are wheelchair users have problems with pressure sores (Shaw and Monahan 1989). This is not due to a lack of feeling but to the lack of ability to shift weight independently.

- **Facilitate social interaction and participation in the therapeutic program.** If the person is able to sit upright and be with others, reorientation into social situations is facilitated. It is also important for participation in therapeutic intervention that the client sit upright, have good eye contact and, whenever possible, maintain a midline stable head position.

- **Increase ADL independence as appropriate in such areas as independent mobility, feeding, and communication.** The upright posture will enable clients to use available upper extremity function to manipulate switches, joysticks, environmental control units, and feeding utensils.

Those with head injuries follow a course of recovery over a period of several years. The evaluation and technical considerations are quite different in the early stages as compared to the post-rehabilitation/community reintegration stage. Therefore, the evaluation for seating and mobility for this population will be discussed in three sections:

- early recovery phase
- acute rehabilitation phase
- long-term rehabilitation or community reintegration phase

Different clients will take varying lengths of time to pass through each phase and, in some situations, they will skip or never reach certain levels of recovery. The categories are meant only as broad divisions and not as absolutes.

Early Recovery Phase

Evaluation

This is often a stage of rapid change. Evaluations for positioning devices must often take place in the acute care facility because of the fluctuating medical status of the client. Throughout the day, there are considerable fluctuations in the level of consciousness, and it is optimal to see the client at both best and worst times before deciding on an appropriate positioning device.

Also during this time, it is likely that the client will be spending many hours in bed. Therefore, bed positioning should be provided along with any chair or wheelchair seating device. It is only through this type of comprehensive approach that the client can hope to avoid postural and structural deformities.

Neuromotor Evaluation

There is no set pattern of abnormal tone in clients with head injuries. In some cases, they exhibit a complete decorticate posture (flexion), while in others there is a complete decerebrate posture (extension). Just as often, there is a combination of the two, with one side being decerebrate and the other being decorticate. There are those who are in total flexion except for one arm or leg, which is in extension.

Persons with head injuries rarely exhibit hypotonicity. If the limbs exhibit very high tone and the trunk has fairly normal tone, the trunk may appear to be hypotonic but in reality is normal or weakened from bed rest.

The tonal pattern can change fairly quickly at this time. A number of persons with head injuries also have a problem with overriding ataxia and tremors which are particularly frustrating when the client attempts purposeful activities.

As with those who have cerebral palsy, a number of abnormal reflex patterns can be present. In people with head injuries, these reflexes are reemerging after normal integration; with people who have cerebral palsy, the reflexes never were integrated. However, the clinical manifestations are similar.

The reflexes which are most commonly seen and which affect decisions about the seating system are the asymmetric tonic neck reflex (ATNR), symmetric tonic neck reflex (STNR), tonic labyrinthine reflex prone and supine (TLRP and TLRS), and the positive supporting reaction. (For a full discussion of the importance of dealing with these reflexes, refer to pages 90-96 on cerebral palsy.)

The main difference that can be noted clinically is that because of the age and previously normal muscle bulk and strength, clients with head injuries are much stronger and it is more difficult to reduce abnormalities of tone.

Orthopedic Evaluation

In the early stages, there are few fixed orthopedic deformities. Orthopedic intervention is necessary only if bones were broken during the injury. With early, aggressive therapy and positioning, orthopedic involvement caused by abnormalities of tone can be prevented in many cases.

There are situations in which the abnormal tone is so strong or the rotational component so great that postural and eventual structural deformities cannot be prevented totally. Assessment of the spine, pelvis, and upper and lower extremities should be completed by the therapist.

Functional Evaluation

In the early stage of recovery, treatment personnel are anxious to obtain baseline information. This will provide them and the family with concrete information about progress over time.

Cognitive deficits may include memory impairment, poor judgment, short attention span, and the lack of ability to generalize. Emotional deficits may include apathy, impulsivity, aggression, and irritability. Perceptual problems create difficulty with eye-hand coordination, spacial orientation, and depth perception. Evaluation of ADL status is also necessary to provide a starting point for intervention.

The functional evaluation should be carried out by a variety of professionals on the acute care team. The seating and mobility specialists must be familiar with the status of the client, especially if powered mobility is an option, because it is often cognitive and perceptual deficits—not the physical limitations—which will keep the client from operating a mobility device safely.

If the client is unable to communicate due to aphasia, dysarthria, or dysgraphia, a speech pathologist must be included as part of the rehabilitation team. Augmentative communication devices, initially very simple and then perhaps more complex, should be considered.

Often, there is a "wait and see" attitude during the acute phase of recovery from a head injury. Both the professionals and the family members, hoping for recovery of total function, are reluctant to think about technology intervention, especially in the form of seating systems and augmentative communication devices. However, the delay of technical intervention may allow the formation of severe orthopedic deformities and, in the long run, create a tremendous rehabilitation challenge.

During this early phase, some clients are not verbally or cognitively intact, and communication can take place at only a yes/no level. But for those who are more responsive, higher-level communication skills should be encouraged with the aid of augmentative communication strategies.

The inability to communicate, even for a short period of time, can lead to frustration for the client and family. In addition, professionals can frequently misinterpret the level of cognitive and perceptual deficits in the absence of means to determine the appropriateness of the client's responses to conversation and verbal tasks.

Technical Considerations

Seating systems in the early recovery phase are considered to be temporary devices for several reasons. Most important is that the physical status of the client is improving, often rapidly.

The second consideration is funding. If the client's funds are used for a definitive system early on, there often are no funds left for a new system when the client is about to be discharged and has a new set of functional and environmental criteria.

Therefore, acute care and rehabilitation facilities are using modular systems that can be modified easily for a number of different clients in succession. Often the wheelchair and the seating components belong to the facility and are loaned to the client only for short-term use.

In the early phase of recovery, components must be:

- adjustable to meet the changing needs of the client day to day and throughout the day.
- durable to withstand the severity of the abnormal muscle tone of adult male clients.
- have orientation-in-space adjustments to accommodate changing needs, including alterations in level of consciousness, resting in the chair, position change for pressure relief, and upright positioning for functional and social tasks.
- able to be fit quickly to accommodate the need for rapid change.

Generally, the seating components themselves can be fairly simple if a successful positioning program is started early. Often a planar system with some lateral supports, a headrest, a lap belt, and a flat seat with lateral hip blocks are sufficient to place the client midline. Positioning of the components in relation to each other and in relation to gravity should be carefully thought through to help normalize tone and provide as functional a posture as possible.

If severe tonal changes are forcing asymmetric body posturing, then customized seat and back components mounted with greater degrees of tilt may be necessary. Recline alone is most often counterproductive in individuals with high tone in the pelvic region because they tend to thrust or slide out of the seating system. Other custom modifications can be created as necessary to provide as midline a support as possible for the pelvis, trunk, and head.

In light of the fact that the client is likely to improve with time, these modifications are best made using commercially available and reusable components or pieces of foam. When the client reaches a plateau, then more elaborate, durable, and cosmetic components can be ordered or fabricated.

During the early recovery phase, the most frequently used wheelchair base is the recliner (Shaw and Monahan 1989). These chairs are often owned by the facility, and clients use the device only until they are discharged, until they have reached a sufficient degree of recovery that the team feels the time is right for a definitive device, or, in some cases, until they become ambulatory.

The tilt-in-space systems which are newer to the market are felt to be the system of choice with people who have head injuries, because the positioning of the pelvis to reduce tone is not compromised with angle-in-space adjustments.

The option of powered mobility is rarely appropriate at this time due to the cognitive, perceptual, and attention problems which persist.

Acute Rehabilitation Phase

After several weeks or months, the client who has regained consciousness and has progressed somewhat is discharged to an active rehabilitation facility. Once again, the rate and extent of recovery are different in each situation. In the rehabilitation facility, the client will again undergo a thorough evaluation, and the technical considerations for the seating system and mobility base will be adjusted as progress occurs.

Evaluation

Neuromotor Evaluation

The components of the evaluation process do not change. The client's physical condition at the time of evaluation in the rehabilitation facility hopefully will continue to show improvement. The abnormal pathological reflexes that dominated in the early phase may still be present, but if progress in treatment and recovery has occurred, these reflexes will not be as dominant a force in the client's posture. The reintegration will allow the seating system to hold the client more easily in an upright and functional posture.

Therapists must also look at any persistent abnormal tone and determine what happens to that tone as the client tries to become more functional. For example, if the client is trying to operate a manual wheelchair and still has high tone in the pelvis, there will be an increase in extension at the pelvis and the person will tend to slide out of the seat every time the person attempts to move the chair.

If there has not been an aggressive positioning program during this phase, the persistence of abnormal pathology and muscle tone become responsible for fixed postures leading to orthopedic deformities.

Orthopedic Evaluation

Persistent high tone, abnormal reflexes, and poor positioning result in postural and then structural deformities. At this stage of the evaluation process, the team must note whether the deformity is fixed or flexible. If fixed, the goal of seating is to accommodate the deformity. If flexible, some correction may be possible. At the least, the status of the curve should be maintained.

Functional Evaluation

During the rehabilitation stage, a greater emphasis is placed on working toward independence. Clients are encouraged to take a more active role in ADL activities such as feeding. If manual mobility is not possible due to the severity of the physical deficits, a powered mobility evaluation is performed at this time.

It is well documented that persons who undergo a severe head trauma sustain cognitive impairment (Brink et al. 1970). As stated previously, these cognitive deficits may be manifested by memory impairment, poor judgment, short attention span, distractibility, and poor generalization.

UTREP staff documented the results of the mobility evaluations of 23 clients with head injuries. The greatest problem observed during mobility evaluations was memory loss. In the midst of driving, clients forgot where they were going and became confused.

Poor judgment and attention deficits, in conjunction with the inability to control anger, also make powered mobility inappropriate and unsafe for some with head injuries.

Additionally, these individuals often have emotional difficulties, such as apathy, impulsivity, aggressiveness, and/or irritability. They do not have the normal checks and balances over their emotions: if they become angry, they may not be able to control the impulses to act. This is a major safety concern, as in the case of one client who became angry during his evaluation and drove his wheelchair at full speed toward a wall.

Visual perceptual problems such as eye-hand coordination difficulties, spatial disorientation, and poor depth perception create some concern, but training and experience seem to overcome these deficits.

During the process by which clients with head injuries are evaluated for potential use of powered mobility, all clients are placed in a powered mobility simulator (Taylor 1986). In this way, it is possible to provide appropriate custom seating and allow the client the best opportunity to use distal hand function to control a joystick or alternate switch. If the client cannot use the hands in a functional manner, alternate body parts (such as the head) are evaluated as possible control sites.

Once the most appropriate site is chosen, the client is given the task of driving the chair under close supervision. Based on the initial driving experience, a decision is made (a) to recommend powered mobility, (b) that powered mobility is not appropriate at this time, or (c) that certain skills should be trained and then evaluated again after a period of remediation.

Technical Considerations
. . . .

The client's definitive seating and mobility system most often is prescribed during the acute rehabilitation phase. Although admission may vary from months to a year, clients usually will have their own systems ordered and fit before leaving the facility.

If clients are discharged directly to home, the selected seating and mobility system often will need to be fit and followed with the client on an outpatient basis. However, if the client is discharged to a long-term residential or rehabilitation facility, the seating and mobility components may be revised as progress occurs. The revisions usually are minor and are made within the available features of whatever system the client has.

Many of the principles of decision-making for people with head injuries follow the same criteria as for those with cerebral palsy. (However, the population's physical size will warrant very strong and durable components.) Therefore, the guidelines proposed for cerebral palsy (pages 109-117) are appropriate for clients with head injuries, and only unique concerns or positioning concepts will be discussed in this chapter.

Technical considerations are similar to those in the early phase of recovery:

- Components should be adjustable to some degree. In the rehabilitation phase, the degree of adjustability need not be as great as during the acute phase. The client's condition generally has reached a plateau of improvement, and changes in tone, posture, and orthopedic status will not change dramatically.

- Systems need to be durable to withstand the severity of the tonal problems of adult clients. Heavy use is also expected when the clients are discharged into the community. Families will include the person in family activities. If the client is transported frequently, the components will be subject to additional wear and tear.

- Orientation-in-space adjustments are no longer always necessary. This is dependent on the level of recovery. Many times a fixed angle of tilt can be used as clients sit for longer periods and attempt to integrate into home and work routines. They may also be able to tolerate an upright posture as the condition becomes more stable.

- The appropriateness and cosmesis of the fit is now a primary concern, although the system should still meet the physical and functional requirements of the client. Its appearance becomes very important as the client and family think of reintegration into the community.

Positioning Goals
. . . .

As with any diagnostic condition, the decision-making process begins at the pelvis. Once the pelvis is well located, attention can be directed toward the lower extremities, trunk, and head.

Pelvis

If at all possible, the pelvis should be held in a neutral pelvic tilt with equal weight distribution through the ischial tuberosities. Planar components which provide a midline stable posture are used with clients who have mild involvement. Clients with a posterior pelvic tilt can be addressed with rigid pelvic restraints (Margolis, Jones, and Benjamin 1985; Monahan, Taylor, and Shaw 1989), anti-thrust seats (Siekman and Flanigan 1983), and a reduction of hip angle to reduce extensor tone.

Wedge seats can be used to reduce extensor tone if it is not excessive. Tight hamstring muscles can be accommodated by allowing the feet to retract under the seat, reducing the stretch to the muscles and thereby reducing the persistent posterior pelvic rotation. If there is a fixed pelvic obliquity or tilt, then it must be accommodated with a custom-contoured system. Of the clients followed in the UTREP study, 39% required custom-contoured seat components while 61% could be fit with planar seat designs.

Commercially available cushions designed for pressure relief can be used if discomfort is an issue, especially under the ischial tuberosities. The seat-to-back angle is best left adjustable, especially if early seating efforts have required an angle of greater than 90 degrees due to extensor tone or lack of full hip range of motion. Added range can be obtained in some cases through ongoing therapeutic intervention.

Lumbar pads may not work well. They tend to push the client out from the back of the chair as opposed to promoting lumbar extension. They also make it more difficult for the client to be positioned well back on the seat.

Lap belts should always be provided. Some clients can be held in the seat with the belt at a 45-degree angle to the seat. A belt mounted at a 90-degree angle to the floor holds adults better. Still others require bifurcated lap belts or a combination of the lap belt and knee blocks or knee abductors.

Adduction spasticity is best managed with flip-down pommels. Fixed pommels make transferring in and out of the chair more difficult. They also preclude the use of a urinal while in the seat and they cannot be easily removed if tonal changes make the pommel unnecessary.

Trunk

Midline posturing is once again the goal. This is especially important in the back because the position of the head and function of the arms are closely tied to trunk stability. A back component which has a planar posterior component with aggressive but thin and strong lateral thoracic supports is frequently used.

Because of the size of adult clients and the strong forces applied to the lateral supports, these supports must be solidly attached to the backrest, and the support should be spread over as large a body surface as possible. The depth of the lateral supports prevents the client from coming forward out of the chair or rotating laterally, and the flat back encourages an upright posture. Optimally, the laterals should swing out of the way for ease during transfers.

If scoliosis is present, then the back component is usually custom contoured or offset. Lateral thoracic supports using the three-point pressure system are discussed in Biomechanics, pages 43-64. Chest belts or panels can be used in conjunction with the back component.

Because these individuals have a clear premorbid body image, their expectations of looking as they used to look are

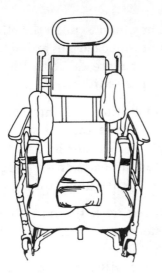

Figure 6.4. Planar back with large thoracic supports offset to accommodate a scoliosis.

very strong. Therefore they are often reluctant to have straps or belts clearly visible. If this is the case, more aggressive lateral supports or anterior support built into the tray can often make the addition of anterior straps unnecessary.

Most often, 90 to 100 degrees is the seat-to-back angle which best positions the client with the least abnormal tone. If the client has difficulty sitting upright for long periods of time, tilt-in-space bases can provide the needed position change while leaving the relationship between the seat and back components fixed. This approach also allows for improvement in sitting tolerance without having to make costly adjustments to the seating system.

Upper Extremities and Shoulders

Contouring of the upper back component can help reduce shoulder retraction. Also, if the origin of the retraction is in a persistent tonic labyrinthine reflex, an upright posture will reduce the effects of the reflex activity and therefore reduce the adduction.

Tray surfaces can position the upper extremities for functional activities and, if accepted by the client, should be kept as small and unobtrusive as possible. Arm troughs can assist with secure placement of the upper extremities for those clients who do not want a lap tray or who have no functional need for one.

Head and Neck

Once again, it is the head that requires the seating team to stretch their creativity. In spite of the pelvis and trunk being positioned in the midline, there are those clients whose heads will not rest in any commercially available headrest.

If post-traumatic visual syndrome is suspected, the client should be referred to a low vision specialist for evaluation. Appropriate prism glasses may position the head in a more neutral position. The head often rests in a position of anterior neck flexion with some lateral flexion. If this is a persistent posture, then anterior forehead components may be necessary.

Flexible bands may not be as effective as rigid ones because clients can lower their heads to get out of them. In a number of situations, the combination of a posterior head rest with an anterior neck support works well to hold the head upright and midline.

As clients gain head control, it is possible in some cases to remove the headrest for part of the day. However, if the client is to be transported while in a wheelchair or tilted in the seating system during the day, then the headrest should remain in place.

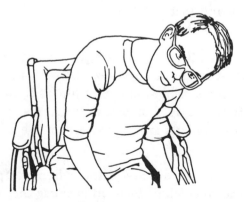

Figure 6.5. Clients with post-traumatic vision syndrome often exhibit lateral flexion at the neck to accommodate visual problems.

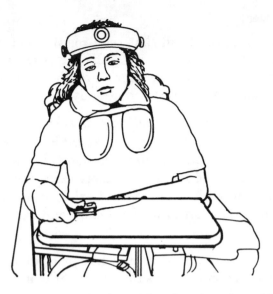

Figure 6.6. A combination of head and neck positioners can provide sufficient stability to allow functional hand use.

Legs and Feet

Accommodation of tight hamstrings can be made by placing the footrests slightly under the seat. The problem with the adult population is that many of the clients are so tall that their feet end up in the front casters. This requires compromises in seat and footrest position and occasionally in the size of the casters chosen.

Many people with head injuries have strong plantarflexion. Placing the feet in slight dorsiflexion can sometimes reduce the high tone. Adjustable-angle foot plates can facilitate this accommodation. Ankle foot orthoses (AFOs) can also help place the feet in a plantigrade position on the footrests of the wheelchair.

The size of the client dictates that, whenever possible, the footrests of the wheelchair be used because they are stronger than most custom-made foot supports. Calf pads and foot or ankle straps can assist in holding the legs in comfortable and relaxed positions.

Long-Term Rehabilitation and Community Reintegration

On discharge from a rehabilitation facility, clients either return home or are admitted to a long-term care facility. Seating and mobility needs should be monitored, but the actual method for follow-up will vary with each person.

A number of service delivery options should be explored, including outpatient technology services and the private sector.

Mobility Base Considerations

Dependent Bases

Dependent bases are appropriate only when there is no potential at all for independent mobility. As discussed earlier, physical limitations can almost always be compensated for by modifications to commercially available powered devices.

Lack of cognitive, perceptual, or emotional skills are the limiting factors in the prescription for powered mobility. If the client does not have the motor skills to propel a manual chair, then a dependent base may be appropriate. They can be less costly and lighter than some of the manual wheelchair bases. In some cases they can be more durable.

Persons who are placed in institutional care can also utilize a variety of institutional chairs that do not fold but which are very durable. Once again, care must be taken not to limit the access of people with disabilities to the community by providing an inappropriate mobility base.

Independent Manual Bases

Manual chairs have a long history of function and durability. If functional mobility is possible using the handrims of the chair or other modes of manual operation (such as tiller systems or foot propulsion), then this is the base of choice. These units can fold to be transported in a car, and seating systems can be easily interfaced with most models.

A thorough knowledge of the market is necessary to prescribe the appropriate size and model. Lightweight models are important for some clients. The chair should be ordered as carefully as the components of the seating system. One-arm-drive chairs or lever-driven chairs can be used for persons who have one arm and/or leg with more function than the other. Care must be taken that the patterns of movement used to propel such chairs do not support asymmetrical postures which could lead to the development of a scoliosis.

For young children, manual mobility devices include caster carts, bicycles, and scooters. A variety of child-sized chairs in colors make the chairs more attractive for the children. A discussion of concepts related to mobility for children appears on pages 33-35.

Independent Powered Bases

If the speed of propulsion is not functional, if energy consumption is excessive, or if the motor skills are not available for manual propulsion, then powered mobility should be considered. Evaluation criteria have already been discussed.

If a client is evaluated as a borderline user, a period of training could be provided before the final decision is made. Also, environmental considerations must be taken into account because most powered chairs need to be transported in vans, and ramps must be built to overcome steps as a barrier to home and community access.

The range of options of powered chairs is increasing rapidly. Children younger than two years of age, elderly people, and all ages in between are being fitted with powered devices. In a study involving 84 children with head injuries at Sunny Hill Hospital for Children (Roxborough et al. 1989), 42 of the children regained functional ambulation. Of the remaining 39 children, 14 used independent manual bases and four received powered bases.

References

Brink, J. D., A. L. Garrett, W. R. Hale, J. Woo-Sam, and V. L. Neckel. 1970. Recovery of motor and intellectual function in children sustaining severe head injuries. *Developmental Medicine and Child Neurology* 12:565-71.

Hobson, D. A., C. G. Shaw, L. Monahan, and C. McLarin. 1991. Anthropometric data for design of specialized seating and mobility devices. A preliminary report. *Proceedings, RESNA conference,* 480-82. Washington, DC: RESNA Press.

Margolis, S., R. Jones, and E. Benjamin. 1985. The subASIS bar: An effective approach to pelvic stabilization in seated positioning. *Proceedings, RESNA conference,* 545-47. Washington, DC: RESNA Press.

Monahan, L. C., S. J. Taylor, and C. G. Shaw. 1989. Pelvic positioning: Another option. *Proceedings, Fifth international seating symposium,* 32-38. Memphis, TN: University of Tennessee.

Padula, W. B. 1989. Post-traumatic vision syndrome affecting seating posture. *Proceedings, Fifth international seating symposium,* 66-79. Memphis, TN: University of Tennessee.

Rimel, R. W., and J. A. Jane. 1983. Characteristics of the head-injured patient. In *Rehabilitation of the head-injured adult,* edited by M. Rosenthal, M. Bond, E. Griffith, and J. Miller, 9-12. Philadelphia: F. A. Davis Co.

Roxborough, L., D. Cooper, M. Story, and A. Stickney. 1989. Pediatric brain injury: Early phase seating and mobility considerations. *Proceedings, Fifth international seating symposium,* 122-27. Memphis, TN: University of Tennessee.

Shaw, C. G., and L. C. Monahan. 1989. Survey of seating providers for patients with traumatic brain injury. In *Proceedings, RESNA twelfth annual conference,* 272-73. Washington, DC: RESNA Press.

Siekman, A., and K. Flanigan. 1983. The anti-thrust secret: A wheelchair insert for individuals with abnormal reflex patterns or other specialized problems. *Proceedings, RESNA sixth annual conference,* 203-5. Washington, DC: RESNA Press.

Taylor, S. J. 1986. A powered mobility evaluation system. In *Selected readings on powered mobility for children and adults with severe physical disabilities,* edited by E. Trefler, K. Kozole, and E. Snell, 69-76. Washington, DC: RESNA Press.

Muscular Dystrophy

Muscular Dystrophy

There are a number of diseases and syndromes which result in varying degrees of musculoskeletal weakness. Only Duchenne muscular dystrophy, the most common and one of the most challenging conditions, will be addressed in this publication.

Duchenne Muscular Dystrophy

Diagnosis

Duchenne muscular dystrophy is an inherited, x-linked disease that affects the voluntary skeletal musculature. Statistics report an occurrence of approximately two to three cases per 10,000 male births (Neen, Beauchamp, and Treadwell 1987). It is progressive and follows a predictable course of muscle weakness.

It is usually detected by the time the boys are five years of age, with symptoms of pelvic girdle weakness resulting in a waddling gait and difficulty in climbing stairs and in assuming the standing posture. The arm muscles are affected later. Muscle weakness begins in axial and proximal musculature, then slowly progresses distally.

By the time the children are about ten years of age, ambulation becomes difficult and requires a great deal of the boys' energy. The need for a wheelchair becomes evident. The seating team ideally should become involved in the management of children with this type of dystrophy just before they are provided with their first wheelchair.

Prognosis

The prognosis for Duchenne muscular dystrophy is progressive muscle weakness leading to eventual death from respiratory or circulatory failure. With spinal stabilization and the ability to provide respiratory assistance with tracheostomies and portable respirators, some people with Duchenne dystrophy are now able to live into adulthood.

Intelligence

Intelligence is within normal limits. There can be tremendous psychological stress on the child and family unit in trying to deal with the nature of the disease.

Medical/Psychological Concerns
- progressive nature of the disease
- progressive orthopedic deformity
- decreasing respiratory function
- sensory status—pressure intolerance when unable to shift weight due to muscle weakness
- increasing depression and the need to control the physical environment

ADL Status

There is an increasing state of functional dependence. Use of upper extremities depends on exact positioning of the trunk and head and learned compensatory patterns.

General Seating Considerations

There is no uniform agreement as to the management of Duchenne muscular dystrophy in regard to seating. Seating management of clients with this disease is determined by whether or not surgical spinal stabilization is performed. Some persons receive spinal stabilization when their scoliosis reaches 30 degrees, and some do not have the option of surgery or decline surgery for personal reasons. In either case, the early goals of seating are the same.

It is with the intervention of spinal stabilization that the seating goals and difficulty of the technical challenge begin to differ. Therefore, the early seating and mobility challenge for both groups will be discussed, followed by the approaches for those with the benefit of surgical intervention and those who follow the nonsurgical route.

A small percentage of clients will develop a stiff lordotic posture due to the locking of the spinal facets in slight extension which deters the formation of a scoliosis, but this may lead to a collapsing lordotic curve which is also difficult to manage clinically.

. . . .

- **Delay orthopedic deformity.** The development of a scoliosis occurs once the children assume full-time sitting or as soon as they stop using the flexible lordotic posture to maintain standing (it compensates for weakness in the gluteus maximus). They also develop hip flexion contractures that are progressive in nature. A midline supported posture can possibly help delay the onset of the postural deformity, but it cannot prevent it from occurring.

- **Maintain independent mobility.** There is a trend to provide these children with powered mobility as soon as they need wheelchairs. This would allow them to keep up with their peers at school and in the play environment. If a powered chair is not an option, then a lightweight manual chair would be appropriate.

- **Maximize function.** A stable base of support would allow the child to use available muscle strength for functional activities.

- **Maintain quality of life.** A seating system should be designed so as to allow the child to be included easily and comfortably in all school and family activities.

- **Increase comfort.** Although comfort does not become a critical issue until the ability to shift weight independently has been lost, it is important from a psychological standpoint that the child be comfortable in an adaptive seating system. It will make future acceptance of technology a little easier.

- **Aesthetics.** It is difficult for these children and their families to accept the progressive nature of the disease, and the addition of any new equipment is often seen as another defeat. All possible consideration should be given to individual choice, and the aesthetic value of any device should be considered.

Evaluation for Seating and Mobility

The complete care of the child with Duchenne muscular dystrophy is the purview of the medical team. The seating team usually is called in on a consultant basis to manage the seating and mobility needs. The evaluation by the seating team is performed to supplement the information already available to the primary caregivers. The process of evaluation will be the same for the client with early or late stage Duchenne dystrophy.

Neuromotor Evaluation

The main problem with this population is the progressive functional loss due to muscle weakness. The seating team rarely does a complete manual muscle test. Of more importance is the functional muscle strength as it relates to the sitting balance needed to propel a wheelchair, manage a joystick, feed oneself, operate a computer, and other functional tasks.

The status of head and neck control is also important. If the child is to be transported in a van, a neck support or headrest should be provided for safety purposes. The motor ability to assist with transfers is important to the design of the seating system. Finally, the strength of the thoracic musculature will determine the amount of lateral support that will be necessary.

Medical/Orthopedic Evaluation

The medical management of this population is done by the primary medical team. In the early stages of sitting, respiratory function is not yet a strong concern.

More challenging to the seating team is the management of the developing contractures. As the child becomes a sitter, the most common contractures are a result of heel-cord tightening which pulls the foot and ankle into an equinovarus deformity. Over time it will become difficult for the child to wear shoes, place his feet on the footrests of the wheelchair, or place his feet flat on the floor for assisted transfers.

The iliotibial bands and hamstring muscles tighten, resulting in hip and knee flexion deformities and abduction posturing. Depending on the philosophy of the primary management team, these deformities will be managed conservatively with bracing or seating or by surgical intervention. The seating team must be aware of any contractures that are present, either fixed or flexible.

As the disease progresses, weakness will result in spinal deformities of either an exaggerated lordosis or kyphoscoliosis. Collapse of the spinal column leads to impingement of the ribs on the pelvis, and pressure sores may result. Also, as deformities combine with lack of muscle mass and deteriorating functional skills, the ability to shift weight independently is greatly reduced. This results in the risk of extreme discomfort and the formation of pressure sores.

Sensory Status

Skin sensation is normal with this population. As long as the clients are able to shift their weight independently, there are no major problems with skin breakdown or discomfort. Once they can no longer weight-shift, they must ask caregivers for repositioning.

Functional Evaluation Results

At the onset of wheelchair use, the child is usually still fairly independent in activities of daily living.

Mobility

During the early stage, walking for short distances can be accomplished with bracing and crutches. Children can assist with pivot transfers and can propel a well-prescribed lightweight wheelchair for short distances. The difficulty is endurance. Although it is possible for them to propel a manual chair, it might not be advisable to use their limited energy resources for community mobility.

With progressive weakness, a powered wheelchair becomes the only option for independence. It is only if the environment is totally inaccessible that this option is not considered. Being able to move assists not only with the obvious ability to be independent, but it also plays a tremendous role in maintaining a positive outlook.

Feeding

Children with Duchenne muscular dystrophy can eat independently during the early stage. Later, small adaptations may be necessary (for example, long-handled spoons). In general, it has been found that this population does not accept adaptive feeding or other ADL devices very well. If they are willing to try an adaptation in the later stage of the disease, mobile arm supports can assist in arm positioning.

Communication

Verbal communication is not a problem, but in the late stages of the disease, the volume will be reduced and the energy expenditure will grow. If the client receives a tracheotomy, speech patterns will change to adjust to the technology.

As the muscle weakness progresses, alternate forms of written communication will need to be developed with creative computer access strategies. In the early stages of the disease, clients can usually use their fingers to access an unmodified keyboard if the keyboard is positioned within easy reach. Mobile arm supports may help when the shoulder musculature becomes too weak to support the arm. Keyguards and mini-keyboards might be of assistance in the later stages.

Transfers

Initially, most of the clients, especially those wearing long leg orthoses, can assist with pivot transfers. As they become weaker and discard their braces, they become dependent on assistance for transfers. Often a urinal is used to facilitate toilet care. When transfers are needed, axillary lifting equipment might be useful.

Although assessment of the child's psychological status is not the responsibility of the seating team, it is essential that the team be very aware of the process of adjustment for the family and child. There will be times when they will be able to deal with changes to the technology, and there will be times when they do not show up for appointments and want no contact with the medical or seating team. There will be times when they are appreciative of the assistance and more times when they might be hostile at the little that can be done with current technology.

As the children enter the more advanced stages, they can become very demanding and intolerant of change, possibly because change often jeopardizes their ability to perform functional tasks. Talking directly to the young men and negotiating with them as adults has proven the easiest route to cooperation in the experiences at UTREP.

Seating Considerations Prior to Spinal Stabilization

When the child first needs a seating system in a wheelchair, the system can be quite simple. The seating can be a modular, planar system or one with slight contours which provides a firm seat and back with some lateral trunk support. It will help keep the pelvis level and the back midline.

Some clinics provide a lumbar roll or support at this stage to facilitate lumber extension with the hope of delaying the development of scoliosis. Research has shown that although posturing in lumbar extension does not prevent the development of scoliosis, it can delay the onset and progression of the deformity by one-third to one-half of the normal rate of progression of curvatures in this population.

The follow-up study also showed that, in those children for whom the progression of the curve was slowed appreciably, the deteriorated state of their cardiac and respiratory systems made them poor surgical risks by the time they reached a curvature of 30 degrees and were to be considered for surgery (Hobson et al. 1983).

Therefore, if surgery is part of the plan, then the spinal stabilization should be done early when the surgical risk is lower and the spine is still fairly flexible. If there are no plans for surgical intervention, then certainly any technology that slows the curvature should be used.

Because of the need to bring the body forward to have gravity assist in the performance of functional activities, it is felt to be counterproductive to tilt the system in space to prevent or delay the development of a scoliosis. The clients usually come forward anyway and lose the lumbar and the lateral trunk support.

If the child is transported in the wheelchair, a headrest is provided at this time for safety. If the legs are pulling into abduction, lateral thigh blocks might be added. The knees should be maintained at 90 degrees, and the feet should rest in a plantigrade position on the wheelchair footrests. If there is an equinovarus deformity, surgical release, ankle foot orthoses (AFOs), or customization of the footrests can be tried, depending on the choice of the child and the preference of the clinic.

A seat belt mounted at about 45 degrees to the seat plane and an optional chest belt should be considered. If used, the seat belt should be fitted so that it cannot be leaned into when the individual comes forward for functional activities. Finally, a clear tray should be provided for those times when a work surface or resting place for the forearms is needed.

There is some controversy as to what type of wheelchair should be provided at the time the child first begins to use a wheelchair. The philosophy at UTREP is that the child ideally should receive a powered wheelchair immediately if funds and the family situation (transportation, attitude) support the decision.

A powered chair would allow the client to conserve energy for educational and social activities. Additionally, he could keep up with his peers in the community, and the psychological impact of his disorder would be slightly lessened. Transportation is often a problem. Usually, however, the school can transport the chair to school and back.

A manual backup chair is provided until the family can acquire a van, for times when the powered chair is not in service, and for the child to propel in limited space situations. The manual chair should be as lightweight as possible and fit the child well in width. With this population particularly, a chair that is too wide will encourage leaning to one side or another; over time, this will encourage the progression of a scoliosis.

If the child is to receive two chairs, the seating system should be able to be placed in both.

Seating Considerations after Spinal Stabilization

The goals of seating following spinal stabilization are outlined below.

- Accommodate the fused spine and the position of the pelvis/trunk in order to maintain the client's balance point for function.
- Maximize comfort. As the boys become weaker, they become less able to shift weight. Most weight shifting is now initiated with the head and upper trunk movement. Sitting in one position becomes intolerable.
- Maintain the midline posture of the spinal column (both fused and unfused segments), including the head and neck.
- Promote upper extremity function. With support of the forearms and careful application of lateral trunk supports, the clients can continue to perform functional activities with their upper extremities.

The seating of the child after spinal stabilization is fairly clear-cut. The pelvis must be maintained in a neutral tilt and must be as level as possible. The degree of accommodation will depend on the degree of scoliosis that was incorporated into the fusion. This can often be accomplished with a planar component or a modular contoured component if the surgical team was not able to obtain complete correction.

At this time, the clients usually use a urinal for toileting, and any cushion should not be contoured so deeply as to prevent this function. It may mean using a flip-down medial thigh support (pommel) or contouring a recessed area for the urinal. Comfort should be a primary concern at this stage, and consideration should be given to pressure-relieving qualities of cushions or materials utilized in custom-fabricated systems.

Thoracic support should support the trunk laterally without inhibiting the movement of the trunk initiated by the head and used for small weight shifts and positioning for upper extremity function. Clients are usually able to maintain the head in the upright position by themselves but should have some head and neck support during transportation.

The hips should be at 90 degrees, the knees between 50 and 90 degrees, depending on the degree of flexion contracture. The feet should rest as plantigrade as possible. Often these clients have tight Achilles tendons which would prevent this posture and require an orthotic device or custom accommodation of the wheelchair.

A tray surface becomes more important at this stage. The child will need it to support his elbows. Often, in the later stages, he will actually use his fingers to "walk" his arm into a functional position for hand use.

Most of the clients have powered wheelchairs at this time. Controls should be mounted for easy motor access. This may mean inboard to the armrest or in the midline which must swing or otherwise move out of the way for transfers. Controls can start with a standard joystick, but alternate controls may become necessary. For example, short-throw joysticks with minimal resistance or mini-microswitch arrangements may make access easier.

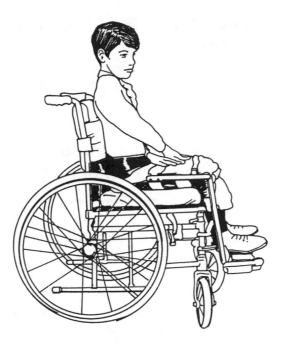

Figure 7.1. Client with muscular dystrophy, sitting on planar seating components.

As weakness progresses, the addition of a tilt system is necessary for pressure relief. A tilt system is preferable to a powered recline both because the degree of pressure relief is greater and the total body posture is maintained during the tilting process (essential with this population due to hip flexion contractures). If at all possible, the system should be powered so the clients can maintain a level of independence.

At this stage, the boys become more dependent in activities of daily living. ADL assists such as mobile arm supports might add to independence but, in general, this population does not seem to have a lot of gadget tolerance. They prefer either to develop compensatory movements to maintain upper extremity function or to ask for help from their care-givers.

Finally, consideration must be given to lifting by the care-givers. Often, as the child gains weigh due to a lack of movement, he becomes too heavy to lift, and a mechanical device must be used. The seating system should accommodate the sling for such a device.

If the individual chooses to have a tracheostomy when independent breathing becomes impossible, consideration must be given to the mounting of the portable respirator.

Seating Considerations without Surgical Intervention

The goals of seating when surgical intervention is not possible are as follows:

- Provide comfortable seating for as long as possible.
- Slow the progression of deformities.
- Provide independence through technology.
- Assist in preventing secondary complications, such as tissue breakdown, respiratory complications, and depression.

Some of the boys with Duchenne muscular dystrophy decide not to pursue spinal stabilization. It is also a regional issue in that some parts of the country are more conservative in the treatments that are offered, and surgical intervention is neither routine nor considered as an option. In these cases, the seating challenge becomes considerable.

As was mentioned, the course of the spinal deformities can differ. A small percentage of the boys (20%) will not develop a severe scoliosis (Gibson et al. 1980). Instead, their spinal facets will lock in extension and they will have a stiff, collapsing lordotic posture. These clients sit longer and with less discomfort than the others. Seating should consist of a midline seat with pressure-relieving characteristics. This can be a custom-fabricated or commercially available product. Care must be taken to allow continued use of a urinal. The back component should provide lateral stability and should follow the contours of the lordosis.

It is often necessary to provide additional anterior trunk support during the later phase of the disease. This can be done with corsets or wide, custom-fabricated anterior chest

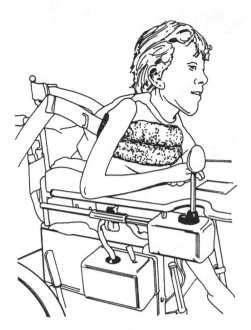

Figure 7.2. Anterior chest supports (flexible or rigid) will often facilitate upper extremity function.

straps (see figure 7.2). Individuals often use this forward position for function, and the anterior chest strap should not interfere with functional patterns of forward movement. Rather, it should provide a surface to lean into, to relieve the weight bearing through the elbows, freeing the upper extremities for function. In general, body orthoses have been found to be poorly tolerated in those with muscular dystrophy.

As the progression of the disease limits functional use of the arms, the client should receive a powered wheelchair (if he does not already have one) if the environment is at all accessible. A manual chair is recommended if family transportation is a problem. Once again, the addition of a tilt system to alter the total angle of the body in space is necessary and should be powered if possible (figures 7.3 and 7.4).

The tilt system becomes critical for resting, reassuming a functional posture, and pressure relief. The nature of the boys is such that they prefer to be in control of body changes

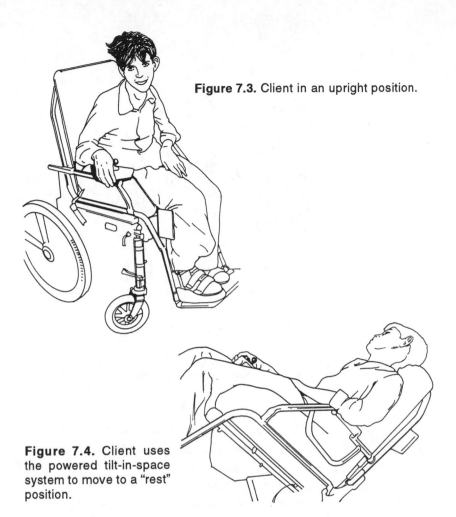

Figure 7.3. Client in an upright position.

Figure 7.4. Client uses the powered tilt-in-space system to move to a "rest" position.

and become very verbally demanding of others if they do not have the opportunity to control their own positions. Therefore, for their own psychological well-being and for the sake of the caregivers, it is best to offer the maximum independence.

The remainder of the children with Duchenne muscular dystrophy develop severe kyphoscoliosis with accompanying pelvic and hip deformities. Uneven weight bearing, ribs impinging on the pelvis, and progressive respiratory problems make sitting very uncomfortable. Seating for these boys must be custom-contoured.

The sitting surface must have pressure-relieving qualities. Several materials can be stacked together to find the most comfortable position. Support for the back must follow the contours of the curves and provide as broad a support surface as possible.

Progression is inevitable. If the progression can be delayed and the ribs kept off the pelvis, then the client will be comfortable for a longer period of time.

Tilt systems are essential so that when the arms are not being used for functional activities, the clients can tilt in space and relieve the effects of gravity on their spines for at least part of the day. Powered systems are recommended whenever possible. Of course, all additional supports (such as lap belts, chest belts, head and neck supports, etc.) are provided as part of the system.

Functional use of the upper extremities becomes less viable as the disease progresses. Some of the older, ventilator-dependent individuals eventually turn to mouthstick use. If this is the case, the mouthstick should be mounted where the client can reach it independently, and switches for powered chairs or computers must be placed within reach. Tongue movement or sip-and-puff controls are other options that can be considered to provide continuous control options.

With this population, the clients will know best what will make them more comfortable. Sometimes the addition of a ⅛″ piece of foam can help them feel comfortable and balanced. Often, if just slightly off balance, they become totally unable to maintain a sitting posture or perform upper extremity skills. Therefore, while evaluating these individuals for seating, it is imperative that the simulation process include a time for them to perform functional skills.

In dealing with the progressive technologies needed by these clients, it is probably most effective to make the appropriate recommendations for change, then do what the client wants as long as it is technically possible and therapeutically sound. In this way, the clients maintain the ability to continue to control a part of their bodies, which is essential to their feelings of self-worth.

References

Gibson, D. A., J. Koreska, D. Robertson, A. Kahn, and A. Albisser. 1980. The management of spinal deformity in Duchenne's muscular dystrophy. *Orthopedic Clinics of North America* 9:437-50.

Hobson, D., F. Desrosier, R. Beauchamp, and G. Martel. 1983. *The spinal support system and other approaches to specialized seating for Duchenne muscular dystrophy patients—A review report.* Toronto, ON: The Muscular Dystrophy Association of Canada.

Neen, D., R. Beauchamp, and S. Treadwell. 1987. Muscular dystrophy challenges for technology. In *Proceedings, Third international seating symposium,* 139-43. Memphis, TN: University of Tennessee.

Spinal Cord

Spinal Cord

More than 11,000 new cases of traumatic spinal cord injury (SCI) are reported each year. The leading cause is trauma resulting from automobile accidents, gunshot wounds, and, less frequently, water-related accidents. Other causes of spinal cord injury or defect include vascular accidents, diseases of the spinal cord such as amyotrophic lateral sclerosis (ALS), congenital birth defects (spina bifida) or extrinsic spinal cord compression, and infections such as tumors or tuberculosis.

This chapter will be presented in two sections. The first section will cover the seating needs related to persons who have a complete or incomplete spinal cord lesion as the result of trauma or disease. The second section will address the specific issues of those who have a lesion as the result of a congenital malformation.

Spinal Cord Injuries

Males sustaining spinal cord injuries outnumber females four to one. Those in the high-risk age range of 16 to 20 account for 80% of the injuries, with a second high-risk age group being between 45 and 50.

Medical Considerations
....

One of the first symptoms to occur following trauma to the spinal cord is spinal shock. This occurs immediately after injury and usually lasts from 24 to 48 hours. All reflexes below the level of the injury are absent, leaving the victim totally flaccid.

It is only as the shock recedes that the spinal reflexes return. There is motor paralysis and sensory loss below the level of the lesion, the degree depending on the amount of damage to the spinal cord. In persons sustaining incomplete lesions, the losses are more scattered and do not follow predictable patterns.

Knowledge of residual motor abilities becomes critical when deciding on equipment needs. Persons with SCI may also have spasticity which can result in hyperactivity of the stretch reflexes. These increase with time, and peak at about one year after injury. Spasticity may also increase in reaction to infection, pressure sores, and even with the time of day.

Other clinical manifestations of SCI can include some impairment to range of motion; dysfunction of bowel, bladder, and sex organs; and a decrease in vital capacity leading to fatigue and repeated minor respiratory infections.

In addition to the direct implications of the SCI, there are a number of related disorders that must be taken into consideration during the rehabilitation of the client.

The most common and often costly result of SCI is the development of pressure sores. The dynamics of pressure sore development are not addressed in this text; this is covered very thoroughly by other authors, and the reader is referred to these sources for information (Ferguson-Pell et al. 1980; Garber 1985; Krouskop et al. 1983; Noble 1981; U.S. Department of Health and Human Services 1992; Zackarkow 1984).

Heterotopic ossification is another, often painful, complication of SCI. Inflammation occurs in the muscles around the hip and knee but can also occur in the elbow or shoulder. Bony deposits or ossification of the muscle result in inflammation and pain with eventual loss of joint range as the person restricts movement. Over time, there is also a loss of functional activity. After about 18 months, the ossification process stops and the client can attempt to regain some of the lost range through therapy or surgical resection.

Respiratory function of clients with lesions above the T-10 level is compromised as much as 60% to 80%. At the level of C-3, the diaphragm is not innervated, necessitating the use of a respirator. Individuals with a C4-5 injury will have some level of respiratory difficulty due to decreased vital capacity. This can result in increased respiratory infections and decreased stamina.

- **Prevent pressure sores.** The factors contributing to the formation of pressure sores in SCI clients are complex. The combination of an appropriate sitting surface (cushion) and a concerted effort of prevention management could help eliminate the formation of many of the pressure sores. Management consists of good skin care, frequent and consistent weight relief, the use of an appropriate cushion, and care to prevent injury during transfers and other activities of daily living.

- **Prevent/accommodate deformity.** After injury, every effort must be made to support the normal body alignment. An active positioning program begun while the client is still in the acute care facility could prevent some of the orthopedic deformities that are seen in this population.

  Spasticity, pain, and the need to position with a posterior pelvic tilt for stability during functional activities will contribute to the development of deformity. If deformities occur, then the goal of the seating system becomes one of accommodation.

  The development of scoliosis is of particular concern in the young person with SCI during growth and with people who have quadriplegia with trunk spasticity.

- **Promote independent mobility.** For people who are used to being independent in society, independent mobility becomes a critical issue. Mobility could be manual or powered, depending on environmental factors and the level of the injury.

- **Enhance functional skills.** The seating system must enable the client to perform as many activities of daily living as possible. A stable pelvis and supported trunk will facilitate the upper extremity function needed to perform many of the activities. Every effort must be made to facilitate independence in transfers, mobility, transportation, and recreation.

- **Inhibit abnormal tone.**

- **Seating and mobility technology** must be compatible with other technologies that the client may need to use (ECUs, desks, and workstation equipment such as page turners or computers).

- **Promote physiological functioning,** especially of the respiratory system. Through supported upright positioning, bowel and bladder drainage and cardio-pulmonary function can be maximized.

Evaluation

Initial evaluation for a wheelchair most often occurs in the early stages of rehabilitation, while the client is still resident at an inpatient facility. Therapists are generally concerned with providing a proper-fitting chair that meets the client's environmental and functional needs and with a cushion to prevent the formation of pressure sores.

Neuromotor Evaluation

A complete motor and sensory evaluation is most often done by the primary treatment team. With SCI clients, the seating is usually done in the rehabilitation facility by the treatment team unless the spinal cord unit is very large and can support its own seating team. The seating team needs to interpret the motor and sensory loss into a functional summary to help determine seating and mobility needs. Table 1 relates motor segments to functional abilities and needs.

As well as determining the extent of the motor loss, the management team must also determine the sensory level. This is extremely important in the prevention of pressure sore development. Persons with incomplete lesions who have the ability to feel even deep pressure in the area of the buttocks are much less likely to develop sores. People with complete lesions at any level are prone to problems.

Table 1
Motor Function by Level of Spinal Cord Lesion

Intact Segment	Motor
C1-2	poor head control ventilator-dependent
C3	weak neck muscles ventilator-dependent
C4	diaphragm intact no accessory muscles of respiration good head control scapular elevators—can shrug shoulders no upper extremity function
C5	shoulder abduction, flexion, and extension weak elbow flexion
C6	good shoulder control radial wrist extension, elbow flexion

C7	shoulder depression
	elbow extension, full wrist extension,
	   wrist flexion, finger extension,
	   minimal hand grasp

C8-T4	good to normal upper extremity function
C8	intrinsics—grasp
T5-L2	partial to good trunk stability
L3-L4	good trunk and pelvic stability hip adductors, flexors, and quadriceps
L5-S1	hip extensors, abductors knee flexors ankle control

Medical/Orthopedic Evaluation

Immediately after injury, the client with SCI is free of orthopedic complications. However, spasticity, muscle imbalance, and unsupported positioning can soon create problems. Almost all clients with SCI sit with a posterior pelvic tilt. This posture provides some trunk stability for functional activities. The problem does not occur until years later when the client is seen for back pain.

Scoliosis is a problem particularly for people with the higher-level lesions because they do not have active muscles to support the spine against the effects of gravity.

Different degrees of hip and knee flexion contractures occur which lead to function losses even if they do not interfere with the seated posture. If the lesion is above the C5 level, lack of elbow extension can become a problem; below that level, clients are constantly using their upper extremities for daily activities, which helps maintain a functional range of motion.

The medical problems of clients who have sustained a spinal cord injury are best dealt with in a comprehensive SCI clinic. In particular, these persons must be careful of respiratory and urinary tract infections, because either can prove fatal.

Although the seating team does not usually concern itself with the acute medical issues, it is wise to suggest that the client pursue ongoing follow-up to ensure general good health, especially since nutrition, weight, and activity level have a direct bearing on the predisposition for the development of pressure sores.

Functional Evaluation

The level of the SCI has a direct bearing on the level of functional abilities that the individual will have. Of course other factors such as motivation, family support, and environmental factors play a role which, at times, can have a tremendous influence on the outcome of functional status. In general, however, the outcome is dependent on the musculature left intact, as illustrated in Table 2.

Table 2
Function Based on Level of Spinal Cord Lesion

Lesion	Muscle Function	Functional Status
C3-4	Neck control Scapular elevators	Control electric wheelchair with head control. With ball-bearing feeders may feed self, turn pages, type on electric typewriter. No sitting balance.
C5	Fair-good shoulder control Good elbow flexion	Dress upper trunk. Self-feeding, writing, typing, etc., with hand splints and/or adapted devices. Assist getting to and from bed. Turn self in bed with arm slings. Propel wheelchair with handrim projections. Needs support to sit upright.
C6	Good shoulder control Wrist extension Supinators	Transfer from wheelchair to bed and car with or without minimal assistance. Self-feeding with tenodesis hands. Assist getting to and from commode chair. Uses posterior pelvic tilt to gain trunk stability.
C7	Weak shoulder depression Weak elbow extension Some hand function	Independent in transfer to bed, car, toilet. Total dressing independence. Wheelchair without handrim projections. Self-feeding with no assistive devices.
C8-T4	Good to normal upper extremity muscle function	Wheelchair to floor and return. Wheelchair up and down curb. Wheelchair to tub and return. Trunk balance but not normal.
T5-L2	Partial to good trunk stability	Total wheelchair independence. Limited ambulation with bilateral long leg braces and crutches. Good trunk stability.
L3-L4	All trunk and pelvic stabilizers intact Hip flexors Abductors Quadriceps	Ambulation with short leg braces with or without crutches depending on level.
L5-S3	Hip extensors, abductors Knee flexors Ankle control	No equipment needed if plantar flexion is strong enough for push off at end of stance.

. . . .

As indicated in Table 2, persons with various levels of motor abilities can functionally operate a manual wheelchair while others will need to rely on powered chairs for mobility. Persons with incomplete, low-level lesions may be household ambulators with orthotics, but often they use a wheelchair for long-distance and community or sports activities. A properly fitting chair that can be maneuvered easily becomes one of the most pressing needs of clients with SCI as they progress through the rehabilitation process.

At times, the experience of operating a powered chair for the first time can have a dramatic effect on clients' attitudes toward all other aspects of life. It is often the first time since the injury that they have had any real control over their lives. Careful consideration must be given to residual motor abilities.

Also important are the projected community needs. If someone who is a marginal manual propeller wishes to continue college, then a powered chair might be the best choice. If there are few community goals, then manual propulsion may be sufficient. Concerns about accessibility, funding, maintenance in rural areas, and the issue of transportation also affect the final decision.

In discussing functional abilities with clinicians, a common comment is heard. With the increase in quality of paramedic and other immediate post-injury care, more victims of SCI have sparing of some components of the spinal cord which can lead to increased functional abilities.

Additionally, the increases in function are not always apparent in the early stages of the rehabilitation process. SCI clients require time after discharge and experience over time to develop their own techniques to solve functional challenges.

Therefore, in evaluating the functional level of any client, it seems wise to defer final conclusions until the person has the time to at least begin to develop functional skills to the optimum. This may mean that technology recommended for persons with partial lesions maintains the ability to be modular. In this way, components that become unnecessary as the client improves can be removed easily to reflect increased functional skill without additional cost.

It is not the intent of this book to provide complete guidelines on the training or technology needed for clients with SCI to be independent in all areas of ADL. However, it must be stated that the higher the level of the lesion, the more important a stable sitting posture is if the client is to have any independence. From a stable sitting posture, added assists such as mobile arm supports may enable increased upper extremity function for activities such as powered wheelchair operation, feeding, computer access, or driving.

Technical Considerations

The technical considerations for the SCI client can be divided into three components: the pressure-relieving seat and, if necessary, the back; the seating system supports; and the mobility base. Careful application of technology in all three will result in an optimally functional individual.

Pressure Management

The first concern regarding pressure sore formation occurs in the acute care setting when the patient is confined to bed. The questions as to mattress choice for the prevention of sores and position change routine become critical. Research has been done (Herszkowicz et al. 1983) into the relative effectiveness of mattress overlays that can provide guidelines for the best choices as well as a format for monitoring for problems.

The literature contains much information on prescription of pressure-relieving cushions for clients once they can be placed in the sitting position (Ferguson-Pell et al. 1980; Garber, Krouskop, and Carter 1978). This section will focus on general guidelines as to evaluation considerations and technology selection, and Appendix B outlines the variety of technical solutions that are commercially available.

Cushions are provided for the purpose of weight distribution to prevent pressure sore formation. They are also useful in providing trunk stability, which helps to provide a stable base for upper extremity function. The type of cushion selected will also have an effect on the ability of the client to perform activities of daily living, such as transfers or sports activities. However, the main purpose is the prevention of pressure sores. A complete preventative program must accompany the provision of any cushion.

General considerations when prescribing a wheelchair cushion are as follows:

- the level of the injury
- hours spent in the wheelchair daily
- activities performed in the wheelchair
- trunk balance
- environment (climate, terrain, temperature, etc.)
- living arrangements (alone or with assistance)
- past history of pressure sores
- body build and sex of the client (slim males are at greatest risk)
- ability to perform independent weight relief
- general hygiene
- wheelchair features (tilt or recline; powered or manual)

The traditional method for evaluating pressure under the buttocks of a client with SCI is with a pressure monitor which measures one location at a time. Although this does provide valuable information, it is only one small piece of the prevention picture. Center of gravity, shear forces, temperature, and moisture also contribute to the clinical picture.

One major drawback to the current method of measurement is that evaluation is not done during functional activities, yet much of the person's time in the chair is spent moving to push the chair, moving forward to reach the computer keyboard, moving for pressure relief, and so on. Clinical tools to obtain this type of measurement do not presently exist, but therapists must take activity level into account when prescribing cushions.

The following pressures are recommended as guidelines with static measurements.

ischial tuberosities	40 mm Hg or less
coccyx	14 mm Hg or less
greater trochanter	60 mm Hg or less
posterior thigh	80 mm Hg or less

The readings should be considered in conjunction with all the other variables that pertain to the individual. Pressure relief of five seconds every 15 minutes is felt to be sufficient to reduce the risk of pressure sore development.

Training in pressure relief techniques should be a part of every client's orientation. Monitoring devices are available to jog memories but, because of cost and complexity, not all clients will have access to these. In addition, many persons with SCI are reluctant to accept any "gadgets" that are not considered necessities, especially if they are generally associated with persons who are disabled.

With more sophisticated evaluation tools, structured teams of professionals working with clients to provide follow-up monitoring, and some excellent commercially available cushions, the prevention of pressure sores should be within the realm of possibility.

However, there will always be clients who cannot or do not come in for follow-up or who do not take the time to maintain their equipment, just as there will be teams of professionals who are not knowledgeable in the best intervention strategies and who tend to prescribe one cushion type for all clients. Thus, unfortunately, there seems to be a continuing population of clients who experience the expensive and debilitating history of pressure sores to the degree that hospitalization and surgery are the intervention of necessity.

Posture

A stable posture has an impact on all areas of ADL. The level of the lesion will determine the amount of auxiliary support needed to provide adequate positioning. It should also be restated that SCI clients, in general, are resistant to technology which is not perceived by them to be essential. Once at home, they will likely take off some of the supports, even if eventual deformity may result.

Functional concerns are also paramount. Thoracic supports which may prevent scoliosis will be discarded if they interfere with upper extremity function or trunk motion used for weight relief.

Sitting postures used when the client is first seated tend to become habit very quickly. If a client is first seated with a posterior pelvic tilt, then it will be almost impossible to change that pattern even if the seating system can provide the added support to the trunk and pelvis so the posterior tilt is no longer necessary for functional activities.

This is also true of those with quadriplegia who learn to hook one arm behind the wheelchair push handle for stability. They are likely to resist giving up the habit. Therefore, caution should be exercised when first seating the client, to provide as optimal a position from the very start as possible to prevent the development of poor sitting habits.

As with other considerations, the level of the injury will dictate the amount and type of positioning the client will need.

Low paraplegia (T-12 or below). Clients with a lesion at this level are independent in the community and require the minimum of seating. A pressure-relieving cushion on a solid seat which may or may not be mounted with drop hooks for removal is appropriate. A seat belt and ankle straps are recommended but frequently will not be used.

Thoracic paraplegia (T1-T10). In addition to the above, clients with thoracic paraplegia might benefit from a slight lumbar roll to prevent a kyphosis. A slight tilt in space of the seating system may provide the trunk stability needed for functional activities without the client resorting to a posterior pelvic tilt. A lap belt may also help hold the pelvis in a neutral tilt.

At this level of injury, a back component is necessary to prevent the development of a scoliosis. This is also the level where the clients tend to be most resistive to thoracic supports or lateral pelvic blocks because these interfere with functional activities. A solid back with midline contours will help provide the stable posture needed for functional activities.

If tolerated, more aggressive lateral supports could be used as well as the lumbar roll. Footrests adjusted with the hips and knees at 90 degrees will prevent additional pressure under the ischial tuberosities.

Wheelchair trays are not often used with this group. Clients either pull up to a table or use a variety of small or stowaway boards if functional needs require a firm surface.

Low quadriplegia (C6-8). A person with low quadriplegia requires all of the support described above, plus a slightly higher back support. The inclusion of a lumbar support becomes more important at this level of lesion as trunk stability becomes more precarious.

Clients are fighting for trunk stability to accomplish functional activities and often assume a posterior pelvic tilt to accomplish this. A lumbar support will serve to facilitate an upright, stable posture with a slight anterior pelvic tilt. It also helps to relieve some of the weight under the ischial tuberosities, decrease shear under the buttocks, and support the low back.

The unsupported low back is frequently the cause of long-term back pain in people with spinal cord injuries. This condition is often considered in conjunction with a slight tilt in space of the seating components to allow gravity to assist in upright sitting. Hopefully, if fit early in the rehabilitation process, the typical posture of the posterior pelvic tilt and kyphotic spine (which a client uses in an attempt to gain stability) can be replaced with a dynamic seating system and a more upright, functional, and pain-free posture.

Clients with this level of injury often can operate a van with modifications and will need as much trunk motion as possible to steer. When driving is not possible (for reasons such as funding), then the independent transfers possible at the C7 level can be useful in getting around. Assistance is needed above that level because the triceps are not functional. Therefore seating components must be removable, swing away, or at least not be too aggressively contoured to allow this level of independence.

Clients with low paraplegia will often use wheelchair trays for functional activities. These can be placed at heights that facilitate individual functional needs.

High quadriplegia (C3-5). These clients have poor trunk stability and will need more aggressive seating components if they are to be functional. If tolerated, the seating should consist of a pressure-relieving cushion which has sufficient pelvic contours to create a stable lateral position for the pelvis. If the client has increased tone in the back extensors, the seat may need to be wedged slightly or include an anti-thrust contour.

The back component should have a lumbar support and lateral thoracic supports. It should be high enough to support the scapular region but contoured so that upper extremity function is not hampered.

The whole system will probably need to be tilted 5 to 10 degrees in order to compensate for lack of trunk control. A seat belt and often a chest belt will be needed to maintain the position. Persons with injuries at the C3-4 level will not be efficient with weight-relief techniques and will benefit from tilt-in-space mechanisms on their wheelchairs. If the lesion is at the C5 level, the client often can accomplish sufficient weight relief independently.

A client with cervical injuries often must wear a halo for a period of approximately three months or until the lesion or surgical stabilization is firm. If the person is seated during this time, the weight of the halo apparatus must be taken into account and the seating system tilted so that the client's already weakened trunk does not have to support the system. Once the halo is removed, the client may be seated in a more upright posture. Headrests are needed with this population when halos are being used and when driving.

Tray design becomes important for people with higher-level quadriplegia. The arms and shoulders need to be comfortably supported. Male clients, in particular, have very bony elbows, and the tray may need to be padded to prevent skin breakdown.

Ventilator-dependent quadriplegia (C1-2). The goal for the population with this type of injury is to facilitate functional activities. All seating considerations described above are still appropriate. In addition, these clients will require headrests, and all wheelchair functions (such as tilt in space) must be powered. In addition, the wheelchair will need to have the ability to carry the ventilator with it.

Several considerations must be kept in mind when seating is done with clients who have this level of quadriplegia. The seating system must facilitate functional activities. The clients will not make compromises in their function in order to have a straighter spine or even to eliminate back pain. Systems must be mounted in the chairs so that clients can enter vans used for transportation.

It will be very difficult to change posture after days or months of sitting. Therefore, it is the challenge of the seating team to provide appropriate support at first fitting or to introduce change slowly while providing sufficient stability in the new design. The lower the level of the lesion the more independent the client can be in the community and the lighter and more versatile the seating and wheelchair components will need to be.

Finally, all clients will need to weight-shift either independently or with powered tilt-in-space units. This is often a consideration when thinking of a wheelchair choice, but it cannot be separated from the choice of seating components.

Mobility Needs by Level of Injury

Level   **Considerations**

T1-L3   The client has the potential to be independent in mobility both indoors and outdoors with a manual wheelchair. These individuals may be very active in their chairs and request individual design changes such as low backs or cantilevered wheels.

C7-8   These clients can operate a manual chair with or without projections on smooth, level surfaces. They will likely have difficulty with rough or hilly outdoor terrain and with endurance if distances are significant. Lighter-weight wheelchairs will facilitate mobility as will any other efficiency measure. The seating system must not inhibit shoulder extension.

C6   These individuals will need powered wheelchairs, but they can use the standard joystick with their hands. They could roll a lightweight manual chair on indoor surfaces, but this would not be functional enough for community mobility.

C5   Functional manual mobility is not possible except for very short distances on smooth indoor surfaces. Projection or coated handrims would be necessary. A recline or tilt-in-space unit would be beneficial to allow the client to perform independent weight relief. However, recliner chairs are harder to push. Functional mobility would require a powered wheelchair which could be operated with the proportional-control joystick.

C4   A powered chair with an alternate control system would be appropriate. The control could be operated by the chin or head or through breath control. Consideration should be given to mounting switches away from the front of the face. An important issue with persons with this level of disability is to look as uncluttered as possible by the technology they require for function.

Proportional control (short throw, mounted behind the head or under the chin) is preferred when possible because of the lesser expense, smoother drive, and less complex electronics. The evaluation team must account for increased neck strength and range which will develop over time when making the decision about the mode of control.

Mobility Needs by Level of Injury (continued)	
Level	**Considerations**
	The decision to choose microswitches that may still prove unsatisfactory after months of fitting should not be made hastily. If microswitches are necessary, the momentary mode, rather than the latch mode, is recommended for safety reasons.
	Sip-and-puff controls were at one time the only option for persons with high-level quadriplegia. They are selected less often now, with the newer ultrasound and infrared techniques that are available. Switches must be mounted securely on the chair. Mounting on the client by way of a bib or anterior chest plate requires very accurate positioning of the client and is vulnerable to movement caused by spasticity and rough terrain.
	At this level, a powered recline unit would be a necessity for independent weight relief. Of course, as one begins to consider powered mobility, community transportation would also need to be considered. Even more basic is the ability of the family to transport the client in an automobile if funds are not available for a van.
C1-3	These individuals are dependent on ventilators. Sip-and-puff or chin switches are most likely to be used. Also, the wheelchair frame must accommodate the tray which holds the ventilator and even the suction equipment. These pieces of equipment usually result in the wheelchair frame being longer than normal, with a wider turning radius. This creates problems in the home and in using lifts for transportation.

Clients with higher-level quadriplegia will benefit from the use of environmental control units (ECUs). Several top-of-the-line powered chairs either have their own limited ECUs or can interface with commercially available units. As technology in voice control becomes more reliable, it will likely be the control of choice for all but those who are dependent on ventilators. Consideration should be given to environmental control at the time the wheelchair is prescribed.

Finally, a discussion about community mobility cannot be complete without reference to the desire of some clients with SCI to drive. Persons with paraplegia can drive with hand controls on a car, as can some clients with low-level quadriplegia. Those with quadriplegia at the C5-6 level will need low-effort steering equipment to drive a van independently.

If a person with lower-level quadriplegia wishes to drive, a thorough evaluation will determine what steering assists will be needed, but it is unlikely that the van will need to be equipped with the full low-effort steering system. Whether driving independently or being transported, all persons traveling in wheelchairs should use safety-approved tiedown systems.

Spina Bifida

Spinal bifida is a birth defect in which there has been a developmental failure of the dorsal vertebral arches to fuse in midline and develop a single spinous process. There may or may not be protrusion of the spinal cord and its membranes through the opening in the unfused spine. The cause of the defect is unknown in most cases, but there is a familial tendency as well as a geographic distribution.

Spina bifida occurs in 0.1 to 4.13 of 1000 live births, but there has been a decline in frequency in recent years. The decline is attributed to genetic counseling and better identification in utero.

There are two types of spina bifida—occulta and cystica. In spina bifida occulta, the defect is a bony one and is not accompanied by abnormalities of the spinal cord, meninges, or nerve roots. The lesion is usually covered by normal skin, and the only visual sign of the defect is a dimple or tuft of hair over the site of the lesion (figure 8.1a). About 15% of the cases of spina bifida are of this milder type.

In spina bifida cystica, the bony defect is accompanied by cystic swelling of the meninges, spinal nerves, or both. If only the meninges protrude, the defect is called *meningocele,* but if the meninges and the spinal nerves protrude, it is called *myelomeningocele* (figures 8.1b, c).

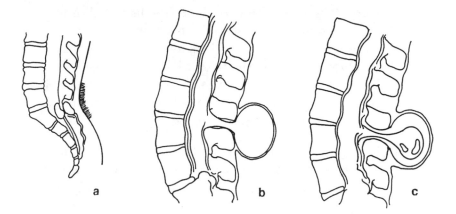

Figure 8.1. Forms of spinal and bony deformity broadly referred to as spina bifida.
  a. Spina bifida occulta.
  b. Bony defect with meninges protruding (meningocele).
  c. Bony defect with protrusion of the meninges and
     spinal nerves (myelomeningocele).

Of the 85% of cases that are classified as being spina bifida cystica, approximately 15% are classified as meningocele with the remaining 85% meningomyelocele. Most often there is early surgical revision of spinal bifida cystica to prevent infection and place the spinal nerves and meninges into the spinal column for protection.

Many persons with this congenital lesion of the spinal cord are able to walk, needing to use a wheelchair for only short periods of time. This text deals with those who require a seating system and wheeled mobility for the majority of the day.

Medical Considerations

- Motor loss below the level of the lesion. There is impaired motor function which can be incomplete; more often, it is complete. The children usually have flaccid paralysis, although spasticity of some muscle groups is not unknown.

- Sensory loss below the level of the lesion. When clients are young, the lack of sensation can lead to skin damage to the feet and legs as the children pull themselves around on the floor with insensitive legs and feet. The lack of sensation is rarely a problem with young children sitting in a wheelchair but does become a problem as they reach the teenage years.

- Weight gain, the lack of bladder control, lack of normal strength in the upper extremities for weight shift, and somewhat passive personalities of many of the children can lead to an increase in tissue breakdown. This tends to occur over the apex of the kyphosis. The skin here is often thin and has little tolerance to pressure due to the surgical repair of the gybus.

- Hydrocephalus is a common side effect of spina bifida. It is an excessive accumulation of cerebral spinal fluid due to blockage which results in a larger-than-normal head circumference and, if left untreated, brain damage. Early shunting of the excess fluid to the abdominal cavity or heart will reduce the pressure of fluid accumulation, although revisions to the shunts are often necessary to relieve blockage or accommodate for growth.

- Neurogenic bowel and bladder. Lack of innervation to the bowel and bladder render them paralysed and nonfunctional. Diapers are usually the choice for early management; long-term programs include catheterization, use of urine-collecting devices, or surgical intervention are chosen depending on regional and family preference.

- Orthopedic deformities. Several deformities in the spinal column are common for this population. At the level of the lesion, there is often a kyphosis (figure 8.2). This is due to both the weakened structure of the spinal column and the weakened musculature which supports the spine against gravity.

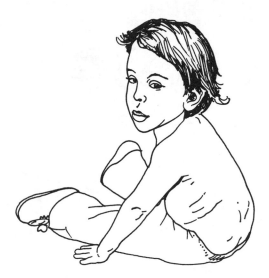

Figure 8.2. Child with kyphosis at the point of the surgical removal of the gybus.

Pelvic obliquity can lead to a scoliosis which is most often seen in conjunction with a kyphotic posture.

Spinal deformities are treated either by orthotic devices or surgical intervention depending on the family preference, the philosophy of the medical team, and the age and level of deformity.

In addition to spinal deformities, club feet (equinovarus) and dislocated hips also commonly occur.

- Intellectual deficits. Children with spina bifida may have intellectual deficits, especially in the presence of hydrocephalus.

- Personality traits. Many, but not all, of these children have common personality traits. They exhibit a superficial but delightful verbal chatter which can mask insecurities or intellectual deficits. They are fearful of exploring their environment and use their verbal skills to manipulate people. Perhaps because of the added weight and difficulty in moving about, these clients become passive (except verbally) in ADL skills such as dressing and transfers.

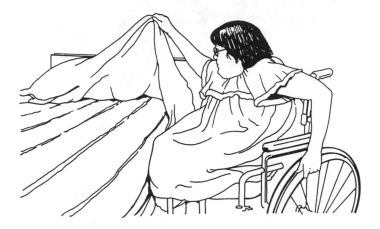

Figure 8.3. Low tone, reduced strength in upper extremities, increased weight, and poor motivation make activities of daily living, such as bed transfers, very difficult.

Goals of Seating

With every diagnostic group, seating and mobility technology must be used as an adjunct to other therapeutic interventions. This is particularly true of the children with spina bifida. Some of the children with low thoracic levels of defects will be able to be functional ambulators.

If the defect is in the midthoracic level or above, it is unlikely that the clients will be functional ambulators in the community, although orthotic devices may assist them to be household ambulators. A thoughtful combination of orthotic devices in conjunction with mobility devices and, when necessary, seating systems, should be considered.

The seating systems and mobility devices discussed here are for children who may be household ambulators but who will need a wheelchair for community mobility. It must also be noted that the upper extremity strength of many children who have spina bifida is not normal, though it is often thought to be. Therefore, although they can be provided with long leg braces for ambulation, they do not have the same clinical performance as the children with acquired spinal cord injuries. They have less energy, less strength in their upper extremities, and, in some cases, less motivation.

Specific seating goals for clients with spina bifida are described below.

- **Pressure sore prevention.** This might be under the buttocks (especially as the children reach the teenage years) or over the area of the gybus on the back.

- **Prevent or accommodate deformity.** Due to muscle weakness, there is a tendency toward sitting with an asymmetrical pelvis. Postural and structural kyphosis is common. Additionally, the children sit with widely abducted hips which should be brought to neutral.

- **Provide trunk stability.** In order to have maximum performance in the upper extremities, the pelvis and trunk should be as stable as possible and still allow for functional motion.

- **Provide independent mobility.** Children need independent functional mobility from a very early age. In order to keep up with their peers, learn from moving in their environment, and prevent the development of passive personality traits, a variety of mobility aids should be made available to children with spina bifida.

Technical Considerations

Early Intervention

For young children with lumbar or sacral lesions, seating technology can be quite simple. A foam cushion that includes pelvic blocks to encourage neutral positioning of the legs, along with a lap belt, is often all that is required.

If the child has a higher lesion, then a seat back and sometimes a headrest are also needed. The back component could be designed to provide lateral stability, but what is most often needed is a contoured area over the gybus. In most cases, it is advisable to design it so that there is no contact between the back of the seat and the gybus itself. If there is any movement at all, the skin is easily irritated. The fabrication can be done so that a larger-than-necessary contour is made, almost like a large cup, over the area. In this way, the skin would not be in contact with the back, but the sensitive area would have some protection.

Custom-fabricated back modules should be made with a double or triple layer of padding over the sensitive area of skin. A second option would be to fabricate a back component that provides contact over areas where the skin is intact and has a hole over the area of the gybus, allowing it to sit into the hole.

Children with very high-level lesions, especially those with hydrocephalus, require a headrest. If the head is very large, it is also heavy. Therefore, children with untreated hydrocephalus should be tilted or reclined slightly so that the spine, which is likely to be supported by hypotonic muscles, is not expected to bear the full weight. Children can develop scoliosis after being seated in a position that is too upright and without sufficient assistance from gravity.

Intervention with Young Adults and Adults

As mentioned earlier, more care must be taken at this stage to prevent tissue damage. Therefore, careful monitoring of skin, pressure readings, and a cushion known to distribute pressure should be provided.

Every effort should be made to design seating systems to encourage independence. For example, smooth surfaces facilitate transfers. Contours should be kept to a minimum for the person who can do a lateral transfer. Sitting heights should be considered for easy access to counters, computers, and sinks.

Mobility Issues

For this population, more than any other, it is important to think about a wardrobe of devices to provide mobility. When a child can walk freely in the community and keep up with peers using orthoses and canes, wheeled mobility is not necessary. However, if the child can move in the home or school but not keep up in the community, then a complement of devices should be considered. A wheelchair or a modified bicycle, for example, is fun for community use (figures 8.4a, b).

For children who require powered devices to move about in the community, manual devices can still be used in the home or school. An exercise program can be established to maintain strength in the upper and/or lower extremities.

The provision of devices does not need to be an "either/or" decision. As with children of normal abilities who have a bicycle, roller skates, and a skateboard, the child with spina bifida should have a choice of devices available for different occasions.

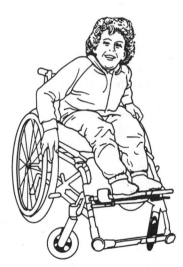

Figure 8.4a. Child using a manually propelled wheelchair for mobility.

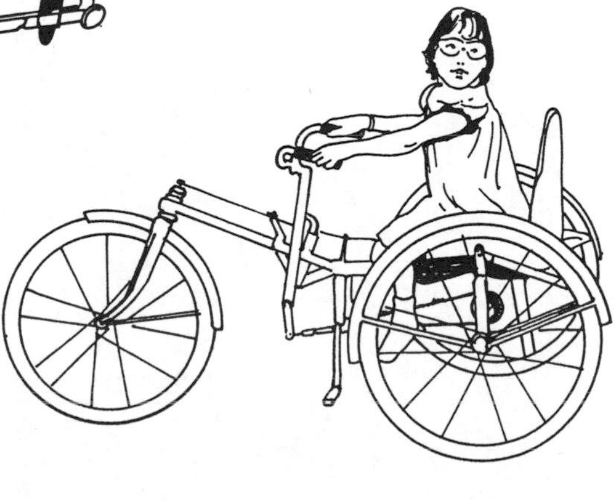

Figure 8.4b. Child propelling a modified bicycle with her hands.

References

Ferguson-Pell, M. S., I. C. Wilkie, J. B. Reswick, and J. C. Barbenel. 1980. Pressure sore prevention for wheelchair-bound spinal cord injury patients. *Paraplegia* 18:42-51.

Garber, S. L. 1985. Wheelchair cushions: A historic review. *American Journal of Occupational Therapy* 39(2):453-59.

Garber, S. L., T. A. Krouskop, and R. E. Carter. 1978. A system for clinically evaluating wheelchair pressure-relief cushions. *American Journal of Occupational Therapy* 32(9):565-70.

Herszkowicz, I., T. Krouskop, S. Garber, and R. Williams. 1983. Pressure relief characteristics of six therapeutic mattress surfaces. In *Sixth annual conference on rehabilitation engineering*, 282-84. Washington, DC: RESNA Press.

Krouskop, T. A., P. C. Noble, S. L. Garber, and W. A. Spencer. 1983. The effectiveness of preventive management in reducing the occurrence of pressure sores. *Journal of Rehabilitation Research and Development* 20(1):74-83.

Noble, P. C. 1981. *The prevention of pressure sores in persons with spinal cord injuries.* World Rehabilitation Fund Monograph No. 11. New York: World Rehabilitation Fund International Exchange of Information in Rehabilitation.

U.S. Department of Health and Human Services. Public Health Service/Agency for Health Care Policies and Research (AHCPR). 1992. *Clinical practice guideline #3: "Pressure ulcers in adults: Prediction and prevention,"* publication #92-0047. Washington, DC.
Note: Phase I, *Pressure ulcer guidelines,* and Phase II, *Treatment of pressure ulcers,* will be available in 1993.

Zackarkow, D. 1984. *Wheelchair posture and pressure sores.* Springfield, IL: Charles C. Thomas.

Elderly Clients

Elderly Clients

The number of people over 65 years of age in the United States is growing. In 1983, there were an estimated 27 million elderly persons (11.5% of the population), a number which was expected to grow to almost 40 million (14% of the population) by 2010 (OTA 1985).

Many of those over 65 are living independently and have no need for seating and mobility rehabilitation technology. As long as health remains fairly stable, individuals prefer to live in the community. However, as people age, a larger percentage will find themselves not able to remain functional walkers, and as mobility is lost, nursing home residence becomes an alternative.

This chapter addresses the needs of those persons over the age of 65 who require seating in a wheeled base for part or all of the day. Researchers such as Bardsley (1989) and Fernie, Holden, and Lanau (1987) have addressed the furniture design needs of elderly persons who are mobile, but the experience of the UTREP staff has been mainly with elderly persons in nursing homes who require seating and mobility assistance for part or all of the day.

Older people reside in nursing homes for a variety of reasons. Many are still independently ambulatory, but some need to use wheelchairs on admission. Approximately 35% of nursing home residents use wheelchairs (Epstein 1980).

Murphy (1989) reports on a nursing home in the Memphis area where, of a total of 180 residents, 105 (about 58%) use wheelchairs, 20 use easy chairs on small wheels designed for attendant propulsion, 16 are ambulatory, and 39 are bedridden. Shaw and Taylor (1988) estimate that there are approximately 600,000 elderly people in nursing homes in the United States who use wheelchairs, or 0.26% of the total population.

People tend to use wheelchairs because of pain, reduced strength or endurance, and visual or balance problems which can lead to falling. As aging progresses, those who can walk with assistance must at some point begin to rely on a wheelchair for mobility.

There are also people who enter nursing homes with preexisting medical problems (such as arthritis, hemiplegia, and lower extremity amputation) which require wheelchair use. Individuals with more severe physical and mental involvement are placed in wheelchairs as an alternative to bed, although the position they assume is often identical to that in their beds.

Some nursing home residents are able to walk but, for their own safety or for the convenience of the nursing home staff, are placed in wheelchairs for at least part of the day. In one nursing home, for example, the residents were seated in wheelchairs to make it easier for the staff to move them from one location to another for various activities, and for fire safety reasons.

Medical Considerations

The body undergoes an aging process which makes comfortable seating for long periods of time extremely difficult. The muscles lose their elasticity and no longer work to hold the spine erect. Muscle mass decreases, and there is an ultimate loss of 30% to 50% of muscle strength (Frymoyer 1985).

The functional and then fixed presence of kyphosis is seen in the dowager's hump (kyphosis in the high thoracic area). Pads of fat under the ischial tuberosities that at one time served as a cushion are no longer there. Additionally, the presence of prior disability (such as CVA, stroke, or polio) becomes magnified as age progresses.

People tend not to shift weight as often as previously, due to lack of energy or mental awareness. Along with thin skin and loss of muscle bulk and fat pads, this can lead to pressure areas developing under the buttocks and/or sacrum.

One other consideration for elderly persons is the potential risk for fractures due to osteoporosis and/or falls. Poor balance, vision, and the use of certain medications can lead to falling accidents.

Seating and Mobility Problems for Older People in Institutions

Table 3 indicates the problems experienced by nursing home residents who use wheelchairs.

Table 3
Seating Problems of Extended Care Residents

Problem Area	Number of Residents Reporting Problems in Response to Specific Questions	Number of Residents Saying the Problem Area Was the Worst Thing about the Wheelchair
Seat discomfort only	17	3
Back discomfort only	1	
Restraint discomfort only	1	
Seat and back discomfort	16	
General discomfort*	—	5
Mobility hindered (standard wheelchair)	19	13
Lack of independent mobility (geriatric chair)	4	
Slides forward only	12	
Leans to the side only	3	
Leans forward only	1	
Slides and leans to the side	1	
Slides and leans forward	1	
Fallen when using wheelchair	10	
Transfers hindered	6	2
Brakes ineffective*	—	2
Footrests inadequate*	—	4
Pressure sore(s) on buttocks	9	

*Problem areas not addressed by specific questions, but reported by residents

Goals of Seating

Mobility

The primary goal of seating is to provide a safe and efficient mobility device. The most common reason for a person in a nursing home to use a wheelchair is for the purpose of mobility. This ranges from the person who uses a wheelchair for transportation purposes only, to the one who uses it as a seating and mobility device, to the one who is placed in the chair for the purpose of being positioned out of the bed for a short period of time.

There are also people who are restrained in wheelchairs to keep them from wandering or falling when unattended. For whatever reason a person uses a wheelchair, the prescription of the mobility device must first meet the individual needs of the client, although it must also meet the needs of the nursing home staff.

Comfort

It is also important to provide a comfortable, therapeutically designed sitting surface. Taking into account the medical implications of the aging process, considerable attention must be given to older persons' comfort in the wheelchair. This is especially true for those who are in their chairs for more than an hour at a time.

Postural Stability

The goal is to provide a midline stable posture, particularly for those clients who have hemiplegia. Because they tend to lean to the affected side, lateral postural stability is a real problem. Also, as a result of being seated in chairs which are too wide, elderly clients lean to one side in order to rest their arms on the armrests of the chair (figure 9.1).

Clients who are elderly tend to have postural instability in the anterior-posterior plane and slide out of chairs. This is due to a variety of problems: the fabric is slippery, the clients do not have sufficient arm strength to pull themselves up,

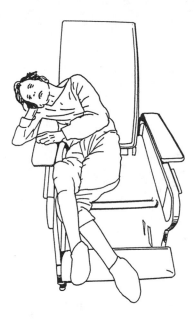

Figure 9.1. The client is leaning to the side in a wheelchair that is too wide.

they have general low tone, or chairs are too long in the thigh length. When kyphosis is a problem, clients tend to assume a long C-curve posture, with their buttocks forward to the front of the chair, in order to obtain support for the upper spine.

Pressure Distribution to Prevent Tissue Trauma

For reasons of comfort and also for the prevention of tissue breakdown, pressure distribution becomes a primary concern of the seating team. This is not just for the area under the ischial tuberosities and the apex of the kyphosis, but also for the sacral area in those who sit with a long C-curve. Thin skin, poor circulation, and the inability to shift weight magnify this problem.

Safety

There are always concerns of safety for persons who are older. Any fall can result in a fracture. Safety issues involving wheelchairs center around brakes not holding, footrests which stick out, and the flame-retardant qualities of the materials used in fabricating seating inserts.

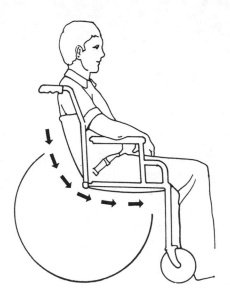

Figure 9.2. Client sitting in a posterior pelvic tilt and thoracic kyphosis.

Ease of Usage and Care

The ease of operating and caring for equipment becomes an issue for those who must be dependent on others for their primary care. If a chair is difficult to push, then residents will not likely be taken very far from their rooms. If directions for care or operation are complex, then not only will residents not be put in the devices properly, but they will also be put in them as little as possible.

Ease of Access

Older persons should be able to transfer into and out of the chair in an efficient yet safe maneuver. If independent transfers are not possible, then assisted or dependent transfers must be easily performed.

Improvement or Maintenance of Function

Well-fitting seating systems and mobility devices should enhance the functional abilities of nursing home residents. They should be able to sit for longer periods of time and participate in activities. Additionally, if they are easily or independently mobile, it is more likely that they will go more places.

Evaluation for Seating and Mobility

People who are elderly bring added challenges for the seating team. Most other clients can be evaluated in the outpatient department. This is possible for the well elderly population who live independently or at home with family members, and for some nursing home residents where transportation is available.

For those who are unable to leave an institution, the evaluation might need to be performed in the nursing home. Also, there will be many times when the client cannot participate cognitively in the evaluation, and information will need to be obtained from the caregivers. This includes nursing assistants with long-time contact with the resident; they are often the best source of information.

Clients seated in unmodified wheelchairs tend to assume a typical posture: the pelvis is rotated posteriorly, the thoracic and cervical spines are flexed anteriorly, and the hips are extended. They also frequently lean to one side. If unsupported, they slide forward in the chair and often are held in only by fabric restraints or seat belts which end up under their axillae. Only a thorough evaluation will determine the cause of the posture, whether it is structural or fixed, and if changes in the seating system can make a difference.

Neuromotor Evaluation

Neuromotor problems in older people are usually the result of pre-existing disabilities. For example, a person who has had cerebral palsy since birth would be evaluated in the same manner as all people with cerebral palsy, with the added considerations for elderly persons which have already been discussed. The same would be true with other pre-existing conditions such as hemiplegia, spinal cord injury, post-polio syndrome, and so on.

Orthopedic/Medical Considerations
. . . .

The primary orthopedic condition seen in this age group is the dowager's hump or high thoracic kyphosis.

The high kyphosis prevents a client from sitting well back in the chair, and the result is a large area of unsupported spinal column in the low back, which can lead to pain.

Many clients who are elderly suffer from osteoporosis which results in fractures, especially about the hips, from nothing more strenuous than taking a step.

Finally, a number of orthopedic deformities (such as reduced range of motion in the lower extremities) can be attributed to poor positioning or posture in the seated position, be it in an easy chair, a positioning chair, or a wheelchair. It is unrealistic with this age group to do anything other than support the curvature. Correction would not be tolerated.

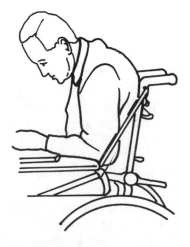

Figure 9.3. Dowager's hump.

Functional Evaluation

Mobility

Possible reasons for the lack of independent mobility have already been discussed. If, in fact, the client is no longer able to ambulate safely for a functional distance, then wheeled mobility becomes the alternative.

The person's environment needs to be evaluated carefully. If the client will be in a nursing home only, with no opportunity to participate in the activities of the community, then a standard, manually propelled wheelchair might be appropriate. However, if the facility schedules outings for shopping, recreation, or other activities, then either a lightweight manual chair or powered mobility should be considered.

Before deciding on independent mobility, especially if it is powered, the client's cognitive skills must be evaluated, both for the person's own safety and that of others in the environment. Also, if the client is to propel the chair independently, then the person must have sufficient energy resources to do so without undue stress or excessive energy expenditure.

The issue of cost must also be taken into consideration. It is often not possible to obtain the most appropriate mobility device because most funding agencies will not purchase wheelchairs for individual nursing home residents. Instead, the home itself provides, from an equipment pool, a chair which may not match the client's needs.

Eating

If nursing home residents are in wheelchairs for most of the day, it is likely that they will eat their meals sitting in wheelchairs as well. It should be determined whether clients will be eating in their own rooms and therefore have a hospital table available, or whether they will be going to a cafeteria for most meals. If they do go to a dining room, then the wheelchair must be able to pull up to a table. Most nursing homes encourage their residents to eat as part of a group in the dining area as long as possible, to encourage social interaction.

Hygiene

Incontinence is a problem for 30% to 50% of the nursing home population. This can result from true incontinence or from not being able to transfer independently to the commode and not having sufficient staff available to respond in a timely fashion.

In either situation, the fabric of the wheelchair seat must be chosen carefully. If the client is independent in transfers, the evaluation should consider the ease of doing lateral or forward transfers in the safest manner possible.

Technical Considerations

In order to define more clearly the needs of those who are elderly in relation to seating, a survey was performed in six nursing homes (Shaw and Taylor 1988). It was estimated that 74% of the respondents had a seating problem. In the survey, 9% had a severe overall problem and required a custom device; 29% in the survey had a moderate overall problem for which custom accessories might be necessary; and 36%, those with a minimal overall problem, could probably use commercially available products.

From the above study, it appears that, for 15 to 20% of the population, custom seating systems or at least custom accessories will be necessary to accommodate the more severe positioning problems. For the remainder—between 85% and 90% of elderly persons who use a wheelchair—seating needs can be addressed with commercially available products. These often are products developed for other populations with physical disabilities (for example, the Jay cushion, developed for persons with spinal cord injuries but which can also meet the needs of older persons).

Seating Guidelines

The guidelines for seating people who are elderly and who use wheelchairs are similar to the furniture guidelines for older persons suggested by Fernie, Holden, and Lanau (1987). The seat of the chair should be low enough so that those who are able to perform transfers can do so safely, yet it should also be high enough to minimize the strength needed to come to standing.

The seats that work best have a small anti-thrust contour (a raised area just anterior to the anterior superior iliac spine [ASIS]), minimal wedge, moderate contouring of the seat cushion, and a firm yet not hard material.

The wedging of the seat will assist gravity in holding the person in the chair against the tendency to slide into a posterior pelvic tilt and forward out of the seat. Wedging can be accomplished either by interfacing the seat component into the frame in the chosen angle, or by actually building a wedge into the shape of the seat itself. The amount of wedging is dependent on the person's transfer technique, because some people slide to the front of the seat prior to standing. The height of this front seat edge also determines the efficiency of foot propulsion.

If pressure is a problem, materials to address this should be incorporated into the seat prescription. Commercially available options that provide good pressure distribution may be sufficient to offer protection from pressure sore development.

If severe deformities accompany the pressure problem, then a custom-formed product probably will work best. Be sure to choose a technique which uses materials proven effective in prevention of pressure areas, or use appropriate padding. Depth and width should be customized to the client for an adequate fit.

There is little information available regarding the selection of pressure-relieving cushions for this population. In a study of 110 elderly clients who were at high risk for developing pressure sores, there was not a significant difference between the group using a simple slab of foam and those using a custom-contoured cushion (Conine et al. 1989).

Another study suggested that foam doughnuts, bare slings, and folded cloth "cushions" produced higher-than-average pressures. However, another study failed to find a relationship between high pressures and reports of seat discomfort

(Shaw, Taylor, and Monahan 1990). This finding suggests that some residents will not complain even when sitting with dangerously high pressures.

The back component should be selected to avoid high pressures over prominent spinous processes. Contouring to provide sufficient support in the low back should also be considered.

If the client is more severely involved, then the seat components will need to be custom-contoured. In many cases, the seat contours will need to be aggressive to assist in positioning the pelvis as midline and level as possible, deep lateral thoracic supports are needed to support the usually kyphotic spine, and there will need to be considerable padding over any weight-bearing surfaces of the back.

Seat-to-Back Angles

A seat-to-back angle of approximately 100 degrees will provide back support without compromising respiratory function. If the client still tends to slide out of the chair, the whole system can be tilted slightly in space.

Every effort should be made to keep the person's eyes level for the purpose of social interaction. (A person who is positioned with the eyes focused at the ceiling will find it impossible to make eye contact with another person.)

Materials

The fabric of the seating system should be water-impermeable if the client has problems with continence. It should be comfortable to the touch, not slippery, and easily cleaned. All fabrics must be fire retardant.

Restraints

The use of restraints or positioning harnesses or belts with people who are elderly is quite controversial. If such devices are to be used, attachment is usually looser than the team would like. This is due to the client's lack of tolerance of the pressure imposed by tighter straps. Pain, poor circulation, muscle atrophy, and just a general dislike of straps could be the problem.

There is also a general reluctance by staff and family to place the client far enough back in the seat and tighten the belts snugly enough to control the person's sliding forward.

Legislation regarding restraints for older persons is also a consideration (Lambert 1992). A physician's order is usually required to restrain nursing home residents. Straps designed for postural support can be included under the guidelines for patient restraint in some instances. As well, family members do not generally approve of restraint systems unless the safety of the patient can be shown to be enhanced.

To be effective in controlling pelvic motion, the pelvic strap should be snug, mounted at a 45-degree angle to the seat, and fit just under the ASIS.

Rigid pelvic restraints such as the subASIS bar (Margolis, Jones, and Brown 1985) are options that can be cautiously evaluated in situations where lap belts and angling the seat and back have not been effective. The rigid devices must be fit carefully under the ASIS and monitored for pressure problems. Generally, these devices are reported to work well if the problem is a persistent posterior pelvic tilt.

One advantage of the rigid restraints is that they cannot be secured unless the client is properly seated in the seating system.

Headrests

If a tilt-in-space wheelchair is used, or if the client is reclined, then a headrest will be necessary. A headrest may also be used to deal with fatigue if the client is to be in the chair for long periods of time.

For those who need headrests, a mild contour is usually all that is required. Positioning the headrest relative to the head is sometimes a challenge. If the client has a marked kyphosis, the headrest is often positioned far forward to accommodate the head position.

Wheeled Base

The choice of the wheeled base should be tailored for efficient propulsion and mobility enhancement. For those clients who propel with their hands, the wheels should be within easy reach and unobstructed by trays or by armrests that are too high.

Chairs with low seat height can help clients who use their feet. Lightweight chairs with low rolling friction wheel bearings will help reduce demands on often limited endurance for clients who can wheel themselves.

If the client needs to have several positions to deal with pressure problems or fatigue, then an adjustable tilt-in-space system might provide some added benefits. A semi-reclining back is useful in accommodating a marked kyphosis.

In some cases, clients are physically and mentally able to manage a powered chair. In these cases, the environment needs to be evaluated carefully to determine whether a large outdoor chair is needed or if a lighter-duty chair or powered add-on unit would be appropriate.

A number of accessories or standard features should be considered.

- Regardless of whether transfers are dependent or assisted, removable armrests are helpful.
- Brakes should be easily reached and must be reliable.
- Leg rests should be swing-away, especially if the client can transfer independently or walk for short times during the day.
- Some clients find a lapboard useful either for postural support or for activities such as eating. These should be easily removed, cleaned, and stored. For clients who propel their manual chairs, the trays must either be narrow enough not to interfere with mobility or be self-storing. With some clients, lap trays can also serve as a means of comfortable and socially acceptable restraint.

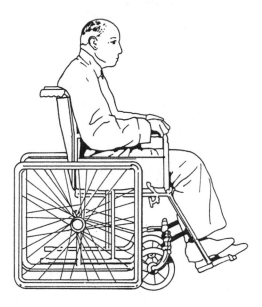

Figure 9.4. Whatever actual technology is used, older adults need to remain independent. Technology must enhance, not reduce, mobility.

Discussion

Three issues somewhat specific to the elderly population warrant a brief discussion: funds for seating and mobility devices, the lack of availability of dedicated products, and the training of those who work with people in nursing homes.

Funding

. . . .

Some elderly people living at home may have private insurance which covers the cost of wheelchairs and seating systems. Those who must rely on Medicare are not reimbursed fully for these devices.

Nursing homes are paid by Medicare/Medicaid for total care and must provide a chair, but there are no regulations as to what kind of chair is provided, or even that a trained professional be involved in matching client needs to available chairs. For cost reasons, nursing homes often purchase a fleet of inexpensive chairs and use Posy belts, diapers, and straps to hold the residents in the chairs.

Fairly simple, low-cost seating systems along with trained personnel can go a long way in ensuring that, even with the "fleet" approach to wheelchair purchase, residents at least have comfortable seating systems that do not add to their existing problems.

Availability of Appropriate Seating and Mobility Systems

A second issue worthy of discussion is the lack of commercially available products dedicated to the needs of older persons. It becomes a chicken-and-egg situation. Commercial companies are reluctant to put resources into products for consumers who do not have the funds to purchase them. At the same time, advocates for elderly persons cannot show available products to the funding agency to demonstrate the value of proper seating.

A very similar situation existed about 15 years ago for children with cerebral palsy. Over time, a range of products has been developed which are now commercially available, and there are a variety of funding options for them. The seating teams must persist with the education of funding sources and the involvement of the industry to promote simultaneous development of both appropriate products and the funding base.

Training

Finally, there is the challenge of education. Nursing home staff, especially nursing aides, need to be trained in the appropriate use of technology. They should know how to place a resident in a seating system and how to clean the seat and the wheelchair, and be able to spot problems (such as skin redness) which should be referred to a professional.

Nursing home workers often are aware of the problems but do not have the skills to find solutions. Efforts are made to improve residents' seating using cushions, pillows, diaper pads, and restraints but, in general, these solutions are unsatisfactory.

Nursing aides typically are minimum-wage personnel with no professional training. The staff turnover is rapid, and there are at least two shifts of staff during the residents' waking hours. Training must be an ongoing process. Instructions must be simple and clear, because many different staff members will be attending to the same resident.

Staff training is costly, time consuming, and sometimes frustrating, but it is essential if the residents are to be able to use appropriately any seating and mobility system prescribed for them.

References

Bardsley, G. E. 1989. The development of a modular system of seating for elderly people. In *Proceedings, Fifth international seating symposium*, 234-36. Memphis, TN: University of Tennessee.

Conine, T. A., M. Lau, S. Massey, and M. Khorassani. 1989. Clinical evaluation of customized foam cushions in preventing decubitus ulcers in elderly patients. In *Proceedings, Fifth international seating symposium*, 237-39. Memphis, TN: University of Tennessee.

Epstein, C. F. 1980. Wheelchair management: Developing a system for long-term care facilities. *Journal of Long-Term Care Administration* 8(2):1-12.

Fernie, G. R., J. M. Holden, and K. Lanau. 1987. Chair design for the elderly. In *Proceedings, Third international seating symposium*, 212-18. Memphis, TN: University of Tennessee.

Frymoyer, J. W. 1985. Musculoskeletal disabilities. Paper read at Toward a Unified Agenda: A National Conference on Disability and Aging, Institute for Health and Aging, September 1, 1985, Racine, Wisconsin.

Lambert, V. 1992. Patient restraints—Improving safety, reducing use. *FDA Consumer.* October 1992, 9:9-13.

Margolis, S. A., R. M. Jones, and B. E. Brown. 1985. The subASIS bar, an effective approach to pelvic stabilization in seated positioning. In *Proceedings, RESNA eighth annual conference*, 45-47. Washington, DC: RESNA Press.

Murphy, P. J. 1989. Aging and ambulation. In *Proceedings, Fifth international seating symposium,* 190-94. Memphis, TN: University of Tennessee.

Office of Technology Assistance. 1985. *Technology and aging America.* Washington, DC: United States Congress/Office of Technology Assessment, OTA-BA 164.

Shaw, C. G., and S. J. Taylor. 1988. Seating for the elderly: A needs assessment survey. *Proceedings, Fourth international seating symposium,* 16-19. Vancouver, BC: University of British Columbia.

Shaw, C. G., S. J. Taylor, and L. C. Monahan. 1990. Institutionalized elderly wheelchair seat comfort. Interim report. *Proceedings, Thirteenth annual RESNA conference,* 117-11. Washington, DC: RESNA Press.

APPENDIXES

APPENDIX A

. . . .

Standardization of Terminology and Descriptive Methods for Specialized Seating*

A Reference Manual
by

M. A. Medhat, M.D., Ph.D., and D. A. Hobson, Ph.D.

Coordinated by
Terminology Task Force of the Wheeled Mobility
and Seating Special Interest Group-09

*This appendix was originally published as *Standardization of terminology and descriptive methods for specialized seating,* copyright 1992 by RESNA Press. Reprinted by permission. For additional copies of this pamphlet, contact RESNA, 1101 Connecticut Avenue NW, Suite 700, Washington, DC 20036.

Introduction

Specialized seating terminology should be completely understood by all personnel involved in developing, prescribing, or applying seating systems. There has been a discrepancy among terms used in different facilities around the world. The need for clarification and standardization of terminology and measurement definitions becomes critically important since specialized seating is such a multidisciplinary clinical activity. In seating, the fields of medicine, therapy, and engineering technology are closely integrated in order to achieve the desired clinical outcomes.

More specifically, when one wishes to describe the seated posture of a person or construct a customized support surface to accommodate an individual's anthropometric measurements, the terminology and conventional methods of both medicine and anthropometric engineering must come into play. For example, in medical practice anatomical locations and joint motions are conventionally zero referenced to the erect standing posture. However, this reference system is limiting when a complete description of a seated person is required, including information on the person's orientation in space. Engineering anthropometry has addressed this problem and has established standardized methods, particularly related to aerospace seating applications. Therefore the approach taken for specialized seating has been to use the conventional medical approach with additions of anthropometric engineering concepts as necessary in order to clarify and permit the complete description of a person's seated posture and the supporting surfaces.

As in any newly developing field the terminology evolves in a rather haphazard manner. At present, the same seating component can be referred to by two or three different terms which can lead to confusion and misunderstandings. Therefore an attempt has also been made to delineate a glossary of the most common terms, complete with a designation as to the clinically preferred term.

RESNA—an association for advancement of rehabilitation technology—established a *Terminology Task Force* within the Special Interest Group on Wheeled Mobility and Seating (SIG-09) to discuss terms and measurement concepts used in seating. The Task Force includes engineers, physical and occupational therapists, orthotists, specialists in seating, and physicians.

The Task Force addressed the following issues:

1. Goniometrics and measurements of range of motion of joints;

2. Anatomical considerations and normal range of motion of different joints;

3. Anatomy and movements of the pelvis;

4. Glossary of anatomic terminology related to seating, including definitions of different deformities;

5. Anthropometric parameters, including definitions of relevant body measurements and orientation in space;

6. Definitions of seating component terms typically used in specialized seating.

The Reference System

The Reference Planes

The four reference planes used to define the position and movement of body segments are shown in figure 1.

Sagittal Plane. Any vertical plane that passes through the body parallel to the median plane (or to the sagittal suture) and divides the body into right and left portions.

Midsagittal (Median) Plane. A vertical plane passing through the midline of the body dividing the body into *equal* right and left portions, along the sagittal suture.

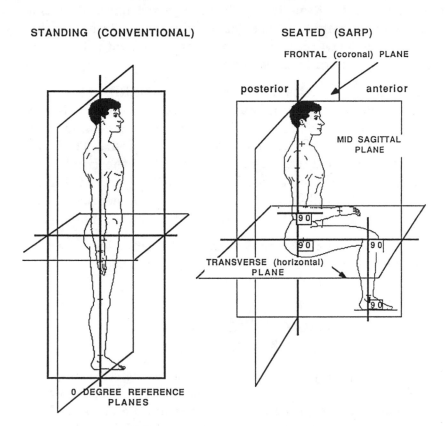

FRONTAL (coronal) PLANE

posterior   anterior

MID SAGITTAL
PLANE

TRANSVERSE (horizontal)
PLANE

0 DEGREE REFERENCE
PLANES

Figure 1. Anatomical reference positions

Frontal (Coronal) Plane. A vertical plane passing through the hip joints and the erect trunk dividing the body into anterior and posterior halves, parallel to the coronal suture of the skull.

Transverse (Horizontal) Plane. A horizontal plane which divides the body into superior and inferior portions. All transverse planes extend horizontally from one side of the body to the other.

The conventional anatomical reference position (CARP) of the body permits description of basic anatomical movements relative to a neutral reference. The individual is standing erect with the head facing forward, arms parallel to the trunk and straight at the sides. Hands are positioned so the palms face forward. Legs are straight in line with the trunk and the feet parallel to each other.

The seated anatomical reference position (SARP) of the body permits description of anatomical movements in relation to a seated reference position. The individual is sitting in a posture that is often referred to as 90-90-N posture. The head is facing forward, the arms are parallel to the trunk and straight at the sides with the elbow at *90 degrees* of flexion and the hands fully pronated. The hips and knees are flexed *90 degrees* and the ankles are in *neutral* position (90-90-N).

Figure 1 also defines the conventional terminology used to describe relative positions of locations on the body.

Anatomical Movement and Its Measurement

The zero degree position is designated as the starting position of each motion. The starting position is comparable to the anatomical position and the arc should be visualized as superimposed on the body in the plane in which motion will occur. The following describes conventional terms for the movement of body segments. Figures 2-4 illustrate several movements in each reference plane.

Flex. To bend a joint in a sagittal plane, around a coronal axis (a line situated in the direction of the coronal suture).

Flexor. Any muscle which bends a joint in the sagittal plane.

Flexion. Bending a joint in the sagittal plane.

Palmar (Volar) Flexion. Bending the *wrist* so the palmar surface of the hand moves toward the forearm.

Dorsiflexion. Bending the *wrist* so that the dorsal surface of the hand moves toward the forearm. Bending the *ankle* so the foot points superiorly (upwards).

Plantarflexion. Bending the *ankle* so that the foot points inferiorly (downward).

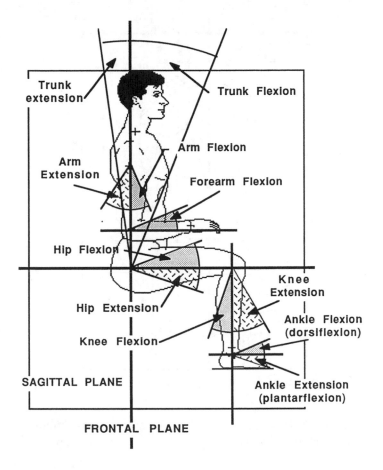

Figure 2. Definitions of basic movement terms (from ASRP in sagittal plane)

Extension. Straightening a joint in the sagittal plane.

Hyperextension. Extending a joint beyond anatomical zero position.

Abduction. Movement *away from* the midline of the body in a frontal plane around a sagittal axis (in the hand a line along the middle digit, in the foot a line along the second toe).

Adduction. Movement *toward* the midline of the body in a frontal plane around a sagittal axis (in the hand a line along the middle digit, in the foot a line along the second toe).

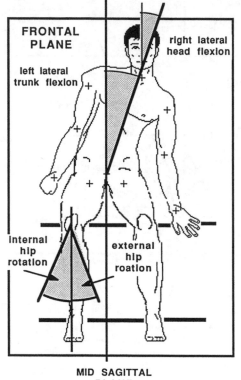

Figure 3. Definitions of basic movement terms (from ASRP in frontal plane)

Internal (Medial) Rotation. Inward twisting movement (toward midline of the body) in a transverse plane around the long axis of the limb.

External Rotation. Outward twisting movement (away from midline of the body) in a transverse plane around the long axis of the limb.

Pronation of the Forearm. Turning the forearm (radioulnar joints) so the palm faces downward (in the SARP position).

Supination of the Forearm. Turning the forearm (radioulnar joints) so the palm faces upward (in the SARP position).

Inversion of the Foot. Internal inward rotation at the subtalar (talocalcaneal) joint in the foot.

220

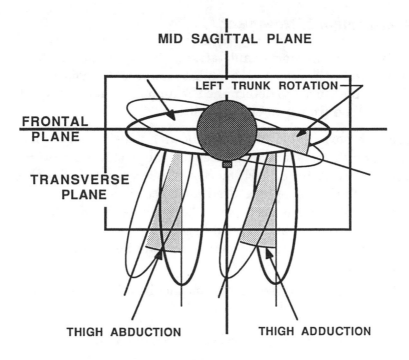

MID SAGITTAL PLANE

LEFT TRUNK ROTATION

FRONTAL PLANE

TRANSVERSE PLANE

THIGH ABDUCTION

THIGH ADDUCTION

Figure 4. Definitions of basic movement terms (from ASRP in transverse plane)

Varus Deformity of the Foot. Inversion at the subtalar joint and adduction at the midtarsal joints (talonavicular and calcaneocuboid).

Supination of the Foot. Turning the medial border of the foot upward so the sole faces inward (varus foot on weight bearing).

Eversion of the Foot. External outward rotation of the subtalar (talocalcaneal) joint in the foot.

Valgus Deformity of the Foot. Eversion of the subtalar joint and abduction of the midtarsal joints (talonavicular and calcaneocuboid).

Pronation of the Foot. Turning the medial border of the foot downward so the sole faces outward (valgus foot on weight bearing).

Measurement of Movement

In describing motion quantitatively, a long bone is like a lever rotating around a fulcrum. As it moves it forms an arc, which is measured to determine the amount of motion which has occurred from a reference position.

Although normal joint mobility allows a wide variety of motions, standardization of the measurement method requires specific definitions of each motion to be evaluated. For this reason, movement is measured as it occurs around an axis perpendicular to one of the three body planes, sagittal, coronal, or transverse, and rotation around a vertical axis. The simplifying assumption is that all motion takes place around uniaxial joints.

Motion of the body segments in the body planes (in the CARP) are described as follows:

Motions in a Sagittal Plane around a Coronal Axis

Shoulder: Flexion and extension, or forward elevation/backward elevation

Elbow: Flexion and extension

Wrist: Palmar flexion and dorsiflexion

Fingers: Flexion and extension

Hip: Flexion and extension

Knee: Flexion and extension

Ankle: Plantarflexion and dorsiflexion

Thumb: Abduction and adduction

Spine: Flexion and extension

Motions in a Frontal (Coronal) Plane around a Sagittal Axis

Shoulder: Abduction and adduction

Wrist: Radial and ulnar deviation

Hip: Abduction and adduction

Foot: Abduction and adduction (midtarsal joints)

Thumb: Extension and flexion

Spine: Lateral flexion

Motion in a Transverse (Horizontal) Plane around a Vertical Axis

Shoulder: Horizontal flexion and extension

Hip: Abduction and adduction in 90 degrees of flexion

Rotation around a Vertical Longitudinal Axis of a Limb or the Body

Shoulder: Internal and external rotation

Forearm: Pronation and supination

Hip: Internal and external rotation

Foot: Inversion and eversion

Spine: Rotation

Anatomical Considerations and Normal Range of Motion of Different Joints

The Spine
. . . .

Atlanto-Axial Joint. Motion at the atlanto-axial joint (the most mobile joint of the entire cervical spine) is primarily that of rotation, up to 45 degrees in each direction or a total rotation of 90 degrees. The zero position is with the person's face positioned directly forward. Since no rotation occurs at the atlanto-occipital joint, rotation of the atlas on the axis will carry the head with it. Approximately 50% of total cervical spine rotation occurs between C1 and C2 before any rotation is noted in the remainder of the cervical spine, that is, between C2 and C7. Slight flexion (5 degrees), extension (10 degrees), and lateral flexion (10 degrees on each side) also occur at the atlanto-axial joint. Lateral flexion is also accompanied by rotation.

Flexion-Extension: C2-C7. Flexion (45 degrees) and extension (45 degrees) occur as relatively pure motions. During flexion each of the vertebrae shifts or "glides" forward upon the one immediately beneath it, compressing the anterior portion of the intervertebral disc, expanding the posterior portion, and widening the intervertebral foramina. The converse of these events occurs during extension of the neck. The greatest amount of flexion and extension is generally in the C4 to C6 region, the area of most stress and strain.

Lateral Flexion and Rotation: C2-C7. Lateral flexion (30 degrees on each side) and rotation (30 degrees on each side) never occur as isolated movements in the C2-C7 portion of the spine. Lateral flexion always causes rotation and vice versa. The intervertebral foramina close on the side toward which the head rotates or flexes laterally, and open on the opposite side.

Motion of the Thoracic Spine. Movements in the thoracic spine (Table 1) are flexion-extension, lateral flexion, and rotation. Total flexion-extension (T1-T12) averages 30 degrees in subjects up to about 50 years of age, declining about 10 degrees during the next 30 years. Total lateral flexion is about 30 degrees, and total rotation is about 80 degrees. As with the cervical spine, lateral flexion of the thoracic spine is accompanied by rotation and vice versa.

Motion of the Lumbar Spine. Movements in the lumbar spine (Table 1) are flexion-extension, lateral flexion, and limited rotation. The average total flexion-extension is approximately 65 degrees, with flexion about 40 degrees and extension about 25 degrees. The greatest flexion-extension motion occurs in the fourth and fifth interspace (fourth interspace between L4-L5 with 25% of the range; fifth interspace between L5-S1 with 75% of the range). Total lateral flexion averages about 40 degrees.

The Pelvis
. . . .

The sacrum is firmly bound to the two iliac bones by means of the anterior, posterior, and interosseus sacroiliac ligaments. It is further reinforced by the iliolumbar, sacrotuberous, and sacrospinous ligaments, and by the lower portion of the erector spinae muscle. Because of this firm attachment the sacrum is considered a part of the pelvic girdle. Some consider the pelvis to be the last vertebra of the spine.

Table 1
Motions of the Thoracic and Lumbar Spines (in degrees)

Movement	Thoracic Spine	Lumbar Spine
Flexion	15	40
Extension	15	25
Total Flexion-Extension	30	65
Lateral Flexion, Right	15	20
Lateral Flexion, Left	15	20
Total Lateral Flexion	30	40
Rotation, Right	40	5
Rotation, Left	40	5
Total Rotation	80	10

Movements of the pelvis occur at the two hip joints and the joints of the lumbar spine, particularly the lumbosacral articulation. Since the pelvis depends on the joints of the lower spine and the hip joints for its movements, it is not surprising that its motion is sometimes associated with the motion of the trunk or spine, and sometimes with the thighs.

Sacroiliac and Lumbosacral Joints. The optimal position at the lumbosacral joint is determined by the amount of angulation that is present.

The *lumbosacral angle* is the angle formed by two lines, one drawn parallel to the ground and the other drawn in line with the superior plateau of the first sacral vertebra. The optimal lumbosacral angle is about 30 degrees in the erect standing position; it is 15-25 degrees in the erect seated position.

Anterior tilting of the sacrum increases the lumbosacral angle and results in increased shearing stress at the lumbosacral joint and an increase in anterior lumbar convexity. When the lumbosacral angle is in the optimal position, the plumb line of gravity passes slightly anterior to the sacroiliac joints. The gravitational moment that is created at the sacro-iliac joint tends to cause the superior portion of the sacrum to rotate anteriorly and inferiorly. This tends to force the inferior portion in a posterior direction. Tension in the sacrospinous and sacrotuberous ligaments counterbalances the gravitational torque and prevents the inferior portion of the sacrum from moving posteriorly. The superior portion of the sacrum is kept from being thrust anteriorly by the sacro-iliac ligament.

The plumb line of gravity passes through the body of the fifth lumbar vertebra and close to the axis of rotation of the lumbosacral joint. Gravity creates a very slight extension moment that is opposed by the anterior longitudinal ligament.

Movements of the Pelvis. See figures 5 and 6.

Anterior pelvic tilt. Rotation of the pelvis in the sagittal plane about a frontal-horizontal axis where the symphysis pubis turns *downward* and the posterior surface of the sacrum turns upward. Increase of the *lumbosacral angle* is greater than 25 degrees (normal lumbosacral angle in the seated position is 15 to 25 degrees).

Posterior pelvic tilt. Rotation of the pelvis in the sagittal plane about a frontal-horizontal axis where the symphysis pubis moves *upward* and the posterior surface of the sacrum turns downward. Decrease of the *lumbosacral angle* is less than 15 degrees (normal lumbosacral angle in the seated position is 15 to 25 degrees).

Pelvic obliquity (lateral pelvic tilt). Rotation of the pelvis in the frontal plane about a sagittal-horizontal axis where one iliac crest is depressed (lowered) and the other is elevated (raised). The tilt is named in terms of the side which is *depressed* (moves downward). A left pelvic tilt means the left iliac crest is depressed and the right is elevated. In the neutral sitting position the line connecting the two ASISs is horizontal. The *angle of lateral pelvic tilt* is formed by the intersection of the line connecting the ASISs and the horizontal.

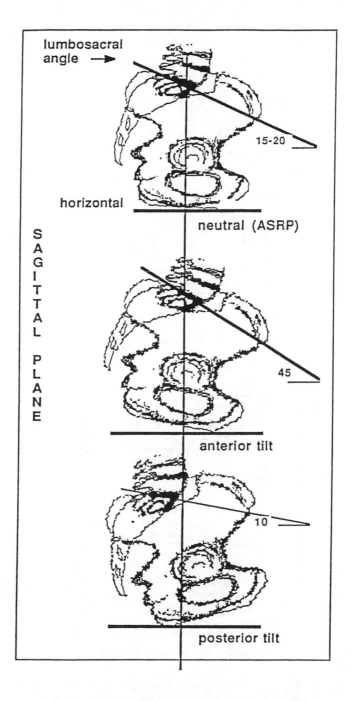

Figure 5. Pelvic movement in the sagittal plane.

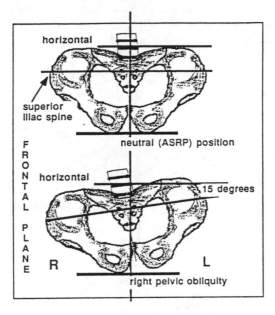

MID-SAGITTAL PLANE (front view)

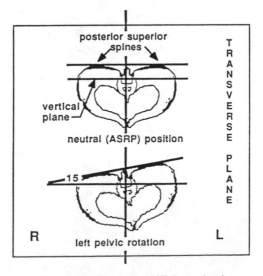

MID-SAGITTAL PLANE (top view)

Figure 6. Pelvic movement in frontal plane obliquity (front view) and pelvic movement in transverse plane rotation (top view).

Pelvic rotation. Rotation of the pelvis in the transverse horizontal plane about a vertical axis. The movement is named for the direction toward which the *front* of the pelvis turns. The *angle of pelvic rotation* is the angle formed between the neutral frontal plate and the line connecting the two ASISs.

The Hip

Hip motions are measured with the person lying either supine or prone. Errors in hip measurement can occur when pelvic tilt is not noticed. The pelvis is in the neutral position when the two anterior iliac spines are level in all planes.

Flexion. Zero starting position: the femur is aligned with the axis of the trunk. Flexion, which is anterior motion of the femur in the sagittal plane, is approximately 135 degrees and is limited only by approximation of the thigh and abdominal wall.

Measurement is taken with the person lying supine on a firm, flat surface with the opposite hip held in full flexion. This flattens the lumbar spine and demonstrates if a flexion deformity is present. The motion in flexion is recorded from zero to 120 or 135 degrees (with the knee in extension or flexion). The examiner should place one hand on the iliac crest to note the point at which the pelvis begins to tilt.

Limited motion in flexion. If the hip flexes from 30 to 90 degrees, or if the hip straightens only to 30 degrees, the hip has a flexion deformity of 30 degrees with further flexion only to 90 degrees (figure 7).

Extension. Zero starting position: the femur is aligned in the axis of the trunk. Extension is limited to 30 degrees as it is checked by tightness of the iliofemoral ligament.

Extension of the hip is measured in degrees from the zero starting position. Two methods are commonly used:

  a. With the person lying face down with a small pillow under the abdomen, the leg is extended with the knee straight or flexed.

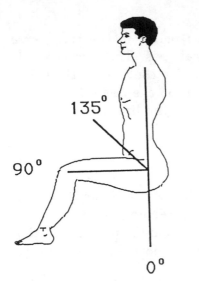

Figure 7a. Hip flexion in seating.

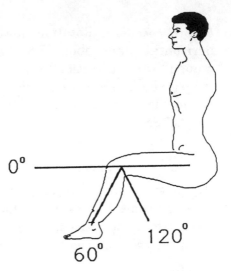

Figure 7b. Knee flexion/extension in seating.

b. With the person lying on his or her back, with the knee of the opposite extremity flexed over the end of the examining table and the hip extended. This is a more accurate measurement of extension because the flexed opposite extremity locks the lumbar spine in position and minimizes movement.

It should be noted that there is an anatomical question whether extension is present in the hip at all. Extension, as seen in examination, is that deviation of the extremity past the zero position and it reflects some back motion. Therefore, it does not measure pure hip extension.

Rotation. Rotation of the hip is measured with the hip in flexion and in extension, and it includes internal (or inward) rotation and external (or outward) rotation.

Rotation in flexion. Zero starting position: measured with the person lying supine, with the hip and knee each flexed to 90 degrees, with the thigh perpendicular to the transverse line across the anterior-superior spines of the pelvis. Because of the orientation of the capsular fibers of the hip joint, rotation is greater in 90 degrees of flexion than in full extension.

- Internal rotation is measured by rotating the lower leg away from the midline of the trunk (laterally) with the thigh as the axis of rotation, producing inward rotation of the hip (45 to 50 degrees).

- External rotation is measured by rotating the lower leg toward the midline of the trunk (medially) with the thigh as the axis of rotation, producing outward rotation of the hip (60 to 90 degrees).

Rotation in extension. Zero starting position: measured with the person lying face down with the knee flexed to 90 degrees and the lower leg perpendicular to the transverse line across the anterior superior spines of the pelvis.

- Internal rotation is measured by rotating the lower leg outward.

- External rotation is measured by rotating the lower leg inward.

Rotation in extension can also be measured with the person supine, with the knees flexed over the end of a table to prevent tibial rotation. With the hip extended in line with the axis of the trunk, rotation is reduced by 30 degrees in each direction.

Abduction and Adduction. Zero starting position: measured with the person lying supine with the legs extended perpendicular to a transverse line across the anterior-superior spines of the pelvis.

Abduction. The lateral motion of the extremity is measured in degrees from the zero starting position, moving the joint away from the midline of the body. Abduction is limited by the median band of the ilio-femoral ligament to about 50 degrees.

Adduction. In measuring adduction, the opposite extremity is elevated a few degrees to allow the leg being measured to pass under it, moving the joint toward the midline of the body. Hip adduction is approximately 30 degrees. The person should lie supine on a firm, level surface.

Abduction in flexion. Abduction can be measured with any degree of hip flexion, but it is usually done at 90 degrees in a supine position.

The Knee

The knee is considered to be a modified hinge joint, with its primary motion in flexion. The motion opposite to flexion, in the zero starting position, is extension. As the motion beyond the zero starting position is an unnatural one, it is referred to as hyperextension. There is a small degree of natural rotation of the tibia on the femoral condyle in flexion and extension. This is difficult to measure accurately. Abnormal lateral motion may be estimated in degrees.

Flexion. Zero starting position: measured with the person lying prone with the knee extended straight. Flexion is measured in degrees from the zero starting point.

Hyperextension. Measured in degrees from the zero starting point with the person lying in the supine position.

Measurement of limited motion of the knee. If the knee flexes from 30 degrees to 90 degrees, or it straightens to only 30 degrees, then the knee has a flexion deformity of 30 degrees with further flexion to only 90 degrees (figure 7).

The Ankle

The ankle is a modified hinge joint, with its primary motion of flexion and extension at the tibio-talar joint. There is a slight degree of lateral motion present with the ankle in plantarflexion. This cannot be accurately estimated. Motions of the ankles should be measured with the knee in flexion in order to relax the heel cord (tendo calcaneus).

A right angle or 90 degrees (neutral position) is considered the anatomical sitting or standing position.

The zero starting position is with the lower leg perpendicular to the thigh (or with the knee flexed to 90 degrees), and the foot perpendicular to the leg.

Extension (dorsiflexion) and Flexion (plantarflexion).
These motions are measured in degrees from the neutral
position. Normal range is 10 degrees of dorsiflexion and 65
degrees of plantarflexion.

The Foot

Motion of the foot is measured in two sections:

1. The *hind* part of the foot (the subtalar joint), and

2. The *fore* part of the foot (midtarsal joints).

Hind Part of the Foot. Zero starting position: the heel is
aligned with the midline of the tibia.

Passive Motion
- Inversion: heel is grasped firmly in the cup of the
  examiner's hand. Passive motion is estimated in
  degrees by turning the heel inward.
- Eversion: motion is estimated by turning the heel
  outward.

Fore Part of the Foot. Zero starting position: the axis of the
foot is the second toe. The foot is aligned with the tibia in the
long axis from the ankle to the knee.

Active Motion
- Inversion: the foot is turned medially. This motion
  includes supination, adduction, and some degree of
  plantarflexion. This motion is estimated in degrees,
  or in percentages as compared to the opposite foot.
- Eversion: the sole of the foot is turned laterally. This
  motion includes pronation, abduction, and dorsiflexion.

Passive Motion
The examiner carries the foot passively through the motions
of active inversion and eversion.
- Inversion: the heel is firmly grasped with one hand,
  while the other hand passively turns the foot inward.

- Eversion: the heel is firmly grasped with one hand, while the other hand passively turns the foot outward in pronation, abduction, and slight dorsiflexion.
- Adduction and abduction: these passive motions are obtained by grasping the heel and moving the fore part of the foot inward or outward. This motion must take place in the plane of the sole of the foot.

Description of Common Skeletal Deformities

Calcaneal deformity of foot. Dorsiflexion of the ankle joint in a fixed position.

Calcaneovalgus deformity. Calcaneal and valgus deformity in the same foot.

Dislocation. Displacement of a bone from its normal anatomical position in a joint.

Equinovalgus deformity. Equinus and valgus deformity in the same foot.

Equinovarus deformity. Equinus and varus deformity in the same foot.

Equinus deformity of the foot. Plantarflexion of the ankle joint in a fixed position.

Genu recurvatum. Hyperextension of the knee; also called back knee.

Genu valgum. Medial angulation of the knee and lateral deviation of the longitudinal axis of the femur and tibia (knock-knee).

Genu varum. Lateral angulation of the knee joint, and medial deviation of the longitudinal axis of the femur and tibia (bowlegs).

Kyphos. Abnormally increased kyphosis (posterior convex angulation of the spine).

Kyphoscoliosis. Structural scoliosis associated with a kyphos in the same area.

Kyphosis. Posterior convex angulation of the spine.

Lordoscoliosis. Lordosis complicated with scoliosis.

Lordosis. Abnormally increased anterior convex angulation of the spine as viewed from the side (hollow back, saddle back, sway back), or the normal anterior convex angulation of cervical and lumbar spine (normal lordosis).

Pes cavus. Exaggerated height of the longitudinal arch of the foot, present from birth or appearing later because of contractures or a disturbed balance of the muscles.

Pes planus. Flatfoot, a deformed foot in which the position of the bones has been altered, resulting in lowering of the longitudinal arch.

Rotational scoliosis. Structural scoliosis; lateral deviation of the spine, with rotation of the vertebrae.

Scoliosis.

> *Functional:* lateral deviation of the spine, both postural and compensatory, which is passively correctable (i.e., mobile). A curve which has no structural component.

> *Structural:* lateral deviation of the spine, with rotation of the vertebrae. A curve which has a structural component. A deformity which is not actively or passively correctable (i.e., fixed).

Subluxation. An incomplete or partial dislocation of a joint.

Torticollis. A contracted state of the cervical muscles, producing twisting of the neck and an unnatural position of the head.

Valgus deformity of the foot. Eversion of the subtalar joint and abduction of the midtarsal joints (talonavicular and calcaneocuboid).

Varus deformity of the foot. Inversion at the subtalar joint and adduction at the midtarsal joints (talonavicular and calcaneocuboid).

Wind-swept (wind-blown) deformity. Described as the triad of:

a. Pelvic obliquity—with the hip on the high side dislocated or subluxated, or with pelvic rotation on sitting;

b. Scoliosis convex to the opposite side; and

c. Flexion, adduction, and internal rotation of one hip (the subluxated or dislocated side), with flexion, abduction, and external rotation of the contralateral hip.

Anthropometric Factors

Orientation or Position in Space

See figures 8 to 11.

Recline. Inclination of the back surface forward or backward. A seat-to-back angle greater than 90 degrees is a positive recline angle.

> *Back recline angle (A1).* Angle between the back surface and the 90-degree reference vertical axis.

Incline. Deviation of the seat angle from horizontal is an "incline." The knees are higher than the pelvis on a positive incline; the reverse would be a negative incline.

> *Seat incline angle (A3).* Angle of the seat surface in relation to the horizontal zero reference axis.

> *Seat-to-back angle (A2).* The angle between the seat and back surfaces.

> *Seat/legrest angle (A4).* The angle of the leg support in relation to the seat surface.

> *Legrest/footrest angle (A5).* The angle of the footrest in relation to the plane of the legrest.

Tilt. The whole seating system is tilted forward or back while the seat-to-back angle remains constant.

> *System tilt angle (A6).* Angle of the complete system in space in relation to the vertical axis. By definition, a change in tilt angle causes an equal change in orientation of each support surface; the seat/back angle, seat/legrest angle, and legrest/footrest angle (A2, A4, A5) remain unchanged. Changes in the recline and seat incline angles (A1, A3) are equal to the change in system tilt angle (A6).

> *Position in space.* Refers to the overall orientation of the body relative to the horizontal and vertical reference axes.

> *Trunk-to-thigh angle.* Refers to the angle between the trunk and the thigh (hip flexion). Sometimes it may correspond to the seat-to-back angle.

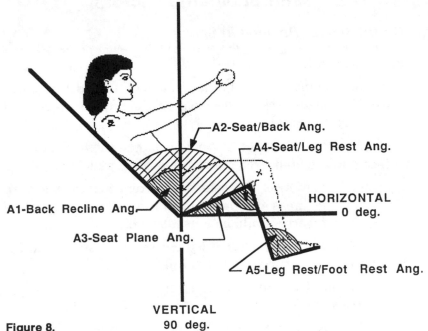

A2-Seat/Back Ang.

A4-Seat/Leg Rest Ang.

HORIZONTAL 0 deg.

A1-Back Recline Ang.

A3-Seat Plane Ang.

A5-Leg Rest/Foot Rest Ang.

Figure 8.

VERTICAL 90 deg.

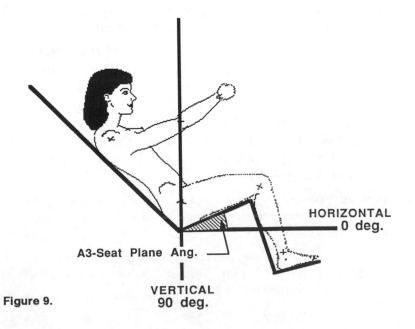

HORIZONTAL 0 deg.

A3-Seat Plane Ang.

Figure 9.

VERTICAL 90 deg.

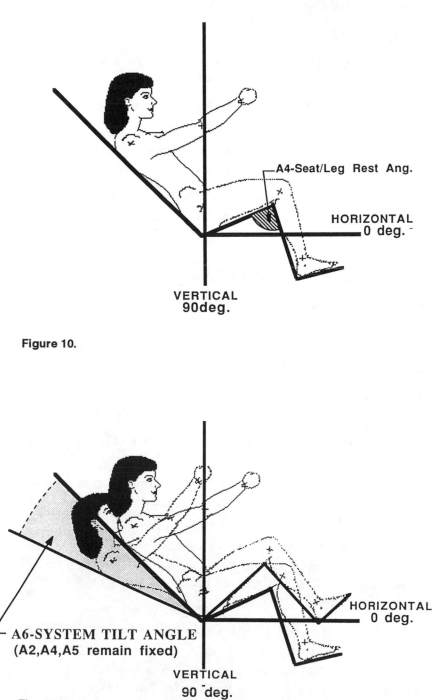

A4-Seat/Leg Rest Ang.

HORIZONTAL
0 deg.

VERTICAL
90deg.

Figure 10.

A6-SYSTEM TILT ANGLE
(A2,A4,A5 remain fixed)

HORIZONTAL
0 deg.

VERTICAL
90 deg.

Figure 11.

Body Measurements
. . . .
See figures 12 to 14.

Sitting height (M1). Measurement from the seat surface to top of head.

Back surface to back of head (M2). Distance from the back surface to the occipital protuberance.

Sitting depth (M3). Distance from the back surface to the popliteal fossa (hamstring tendons).

Leg length (M4). Distance from the popliteal fossa to the bottom of the heel, or the weight-bearing surface of the foot if the ankle cannot be brought to the anatomical position; or to the footrest surface.

Foot length (M5). Overall foot/shoe length.

Shoulder width (M6). Maximum width of the shoulders between the tips of the two acromion processes.

Chest width (M7). Width of the chest taken at the nipple line or the costal end of the fourth rib.

Waist width (M8). Measured at halfway between the lower margin of the rib cage and iliac crest.

Pelvic width (M9). Measured at the level of the greater trochanters.

Knee width (M10). Maximum outside dimension across the knees with the hip joint in neutral abduction/adduction and rotation with the hips flexed.

Occipital protuberance to center line (M11). In scoliosis, the center line is described by a vertical line on the sagittal plane passing through the midpoint of the pelvis (just in front of S2 vertebra).

Acromion height L/R (M12). Seat surface to each acromion (left and right side).

Overall width (M13). Maximum width occupied by the individual. For a person with a fixed spinal deformity this may be from the outer side of one knee to the opposite shoulder.

DEFINITIONS - LINEAR MEASUREMENTS

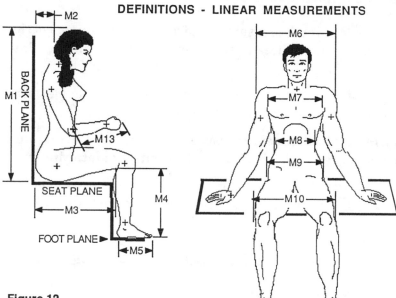

Figure 12.

Figure 13.

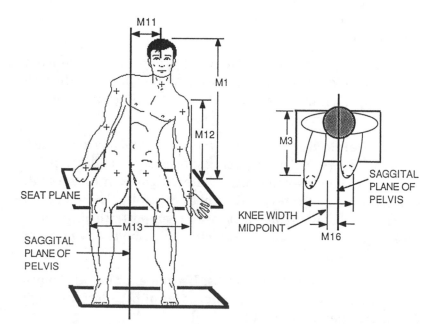

Figure 14.

. . . .

Seat depth. Linear measurement from the intersection of the seat and back surfaces to the front edge of the sitting platform.

Seat width. Linear measurement of the sitting platform from one lateral border to the other.

Footrest height. Linear measurement from the footrest surface to the top of the front edge of the sitting platform.

Back height. Linear measurement from the intersection of the seat and back surfaces to the top of the back surface.

Glossary of Component Terms

Pelvic and Thigh Control
. . . .

Medial Thigh Support. *Synonyms: hip abductor, pommel, anti-adductor pad, abductor post, abductor wedge, knee abductor.* Maintains the hips of the seated individual in a prescribed amount of abduction, or prevents adduction of the hips (figure 15).

Lateral Thigh Support. *Synonyms: lateral knee adductor, adduction pads.* Prevents excessive or unwanted abduction of the hips, or provides a counterpoint for control of hip external rotation (figure 15).

Lateral Pelvic Support. *Synonyms: hip support pads, lateral hip blocks, pelvic support, side cushions, hip guides.* Maintains the hips/pelvis in a centered position in the seat, and provides a counterpoint to help control pelvic obliquity in conjunction with lateral thoracic support. In some systems, the pads can be constructed to provide support for armrests (figure 15).

Lateral Pelvic/Thigh Supports. If pads are the full length of the seat, they can serve the purposes of both lateral thigh and lateral pelvic supports.

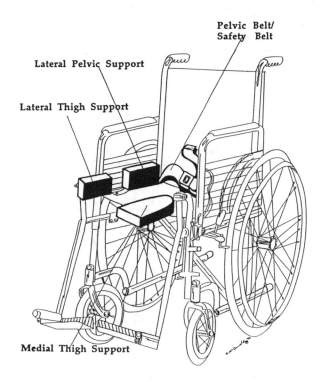

Pelvic Belt/
Safety Belt

Lateral Pelvic Support

Lateral Thigh Support

Medial Thigh Support

Figure 15.

Anterior Pelvic Support

Pelvic stabilizer provides an anterior point of control at the symphysis pubis to maintain the pelvis in an upright position; it can be designed to be used as a hip abductor.

ASIS Pads/Bar Pelvic Positioners. *Synonym: anterior pelvic bar.* Provides an anterior point for pelvic control at one or both anterior superior iliac spines to maintain the pelvis in an upright position or to prevent pelvic rotation or obliquity. Positioned *inferior* to the ASISs (figure 16).

Pelvic Belt. *Synonyms: hip belt, hip strap.* Crosses the hip joints at the anterior joint crease and interior to the ASIS. Controls extensor thrust at the hips, and to a lesser extent, controls the pelvic position. It should be noted that a pelvic belt can be placed at a 45 to 90 degree angle in relation to the seat. A pelvic belt can be combined with a safety belt (figure 15).

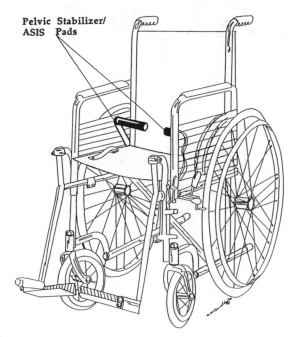

Pelvic Stabilizer/
ASIS Pads

Figure 16.

Safety Belt. *Synonym: lap belt.* Prevents accidental forward movement out of the seating system; does not control the pelvis.

Trunk Control Components

Lateral Thoracic Supports. *Synonyms: scoliosis pads, lateral trunk pads, trunk control system.* Provides lateral support to the thoracic spine; when contoured, they can provide anterior and/or posterior support as well (figure 17).

Posterior Lumbar Support. *Synonyms: lumbar roll/bar.* Provides posterior support for the lumbar curve (figure 17).

Sacral Support. Provides posterior support to the pelvis.

Anterior Trunk Support
- Chest Strap/Chest Piece (Harness): *Synonyms: chest belt, chest strap, chest panel, butterfly harness.* Provides anterior upper trunk control, and controls kyphotic posture (figures 18, 19).

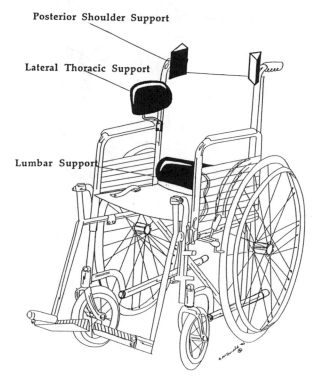

Posterior Shoulder Support

Lateral Thoracic Support

Lumbar Support

Figure 17.

- Rigid Tray Mounted Anterior Trunk Support provides anterior trunk control when tray is in place.

Shoulder Control Components

Posterior Shoulder Support. *Synonyms: shoulder protractors, scapular bars, protraction pads, elbow blocks.* Encourages scapular abduction (movement away from the midline of the body) with concurrent midline position of the upper extremities to improve upper extremity function (figure 17).

Anterior Shoulder Support. *Synonyms: shoulder retractors, wishbone piece, cow-horns.* Retracts the shoulders (backward movement); provides upper trunk control, and controls kyphotic posture of the spine (figure 18).

Superior Shoulder Support. Depresses elevated shoulders.

Anterior Shoulder Supports

Anterior Trunk Support:

Chest Strap

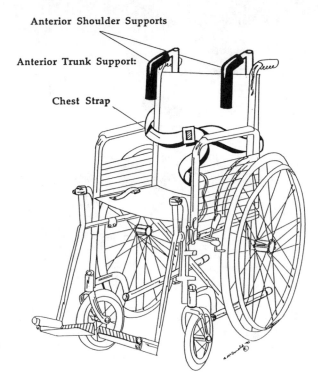

Figure 18.

Chest Harness

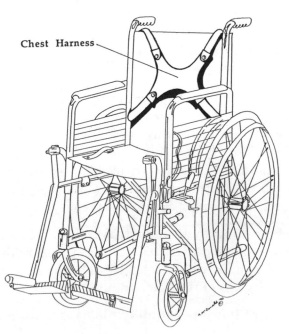

Figure 19.

Head and Neck Control Components

Posterior Neck Support. *Synonyms: neck collar, neckrest.* Provides support to the cervical spine; fits below the occiput (figure 20).

Posterior Head Support. *Synonym: headrest.* Provides posterior support to the head. Can be used to prevent whiplash injury or for head control during transportation (figure 20).

Lateral Head Support. Prevents lateral rotation or lateral flexion of the neck.

Anterior Head Support. *Synonyms: forehead band, halo, head strap, head band.* Provides an anterior stop to forward head drop.

Circumferential Head and Neck Support. *Synonyms: cervical collar, C-collar.* Provides head support to head and neck with a padded collar around the neck (figure 20).

Upper Extremity Control Components

Arm Support. *Synonym: armrest.* Support surface for forearm (figure 21).

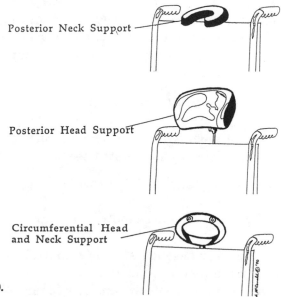

Posterior Neck Support

Posterior Head Support

Circumferential Head and Neck Support

Figure 20.

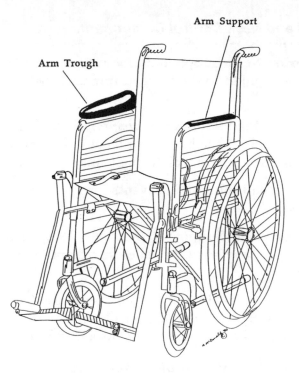

Arm Support

Arm Trough

Figure 21.

Arm Trough. Forearm surface with lateral and posterior support (figure 21).

Tray. *Synonyms: anterior upper extremity support surface, lap tray; lapboard; arm restraint tray.* Provides support to the arms and upper extremities, and can be used to assist in upper trunk positioning or upper extremity positioning. Can be horizontal or angled (figure 22).

Lower Extremity Control Components
. . . .

Posterior Calf Support. *Synonyms: legrest, calf panel.* Provides support to the lower leg and limits knee flexion (figure 23).

Foot Support. *Synonym: footrest.* Provides support under the feet.
- Foot Platform is a one-piece footrest to support both feet.
- Foot Channel provides medial/lateral control as well as support underneath the feet.
- Foot Plates are individual foot supports (figure 23).

Tray (Anterior Upper Extremity
Support Surface)

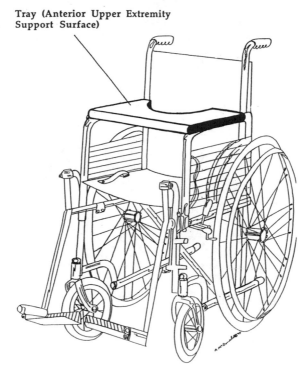

Figure 22.

Foot Positioner

- Posterior Heel Support (*Synonyms: heel loop, heel cup*) is a curved or flat support behind the heel (figure 23).
- Ankle Strap maintains foot against posterior heel support with strap crossing neutral ankle at a 45-degree line of pull (figure 24).
- Toe Strap (*Synonym: midfoot strap*) provides a line of pull over the ball of the foot to control dorsiflexion or forefoot movement.
- Shoe Holder provides the same support as the posterior heel support, ankle straps, and toe straps.

Anterior Knee Support. Provides restraint at the knee joints to help stabilize the pelvis. Can be used to prevent the person sliding forward and, when contoured, limits the amount of hip abduction and adduction (figure 24).

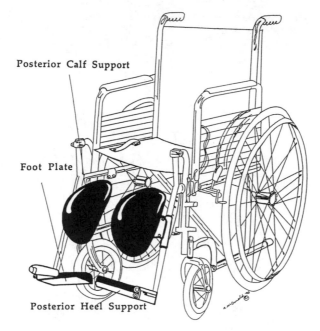

Posterior Calf Support

Foot Plate

Posterior Heel Support

Figure 23.

Anterior Leg Support. Provides anterior support to the lower leg to help stabilize the pelvis or prevent excessive leg extension.

Seat and Back Terms

Firm Back/Solid Back Insert. *Synonyms: solid back, drop back, adjustable depth back.* Designed to fit between or in front of the back uprights of the wheelchair frame to provide back support and allow the adjustment of seat depth.

Firm Seat/Solid Seat Insert. *Synonyms: solid seat, solid seat insert, drop seat.* Designed to fit between or on top of the seat rails of the wheelchair frame to provide a firm sitting platform, and allow angle of the sitting platform.

Planar Seat/Back. Seating system with flat seat and back surfaces, usually upholstered and padded with foam. These systems are very adjustable and have many modular components that can be combined for an individual's specific needs.

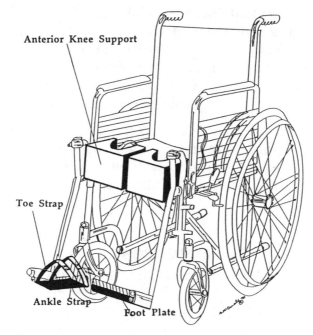

Anterior Knee Support

Toe Strap

Ankle Strap

Foot Plate

Figure 24.

Prefabricated components are available from many companies, or custom components can be fabricated from foam and plywood.

Contoured Seat/Back. Seating system with contoured shaping to conform to body parts for increased pressure distribution or posture control. Prefabricated systems are available with slight contouring. Custom contoured seats can be made by making a mold of the individual in the desired position and using the mold to fabricate a seat.

Summary Discussion

It is realized that the Standardized Terminology and recommended practices presented above are only a beginning. The material has been presented at three professional meetings, two in North America and one in the United Kingdom, for discussion and critique. The resulting critiques plus those given by members of the RESNA Special Interest Group on

Wheeled Mobility and Seating (SIG-09) have been invaluable throughout the refinement process. It is hoped that this publication will in turn engender continued comments and suggestions so that continued refinements may take place. The authors and the RESNA Task Force will be most receptive to further constructive suggestions for improvement.

The long-term goal is to establish accepted terminology and descriptive methods that can provide an additional building block upon which the field of specialized seating and mobility can grow and mature into a fully accepted research and clinical endeavor.

References

American Medical Association. Committee on Rating of Mental and Physical Impairment. 1977. *Guides to the evaluation of permanent impairment.* Chicago: AMA.

Cooperman, D. R., E. Bartucci, E. Dietrick, and E. Miller. 1987. Hip dislocation in spastic cerebral palsy. *Journal of Pediatric Orthopedics* 7:268-76.

Dorland's illustrated medical dictionary. 1974. Philadelphia: W. B. Saunders.

Gerhardt, J. J., P. S. King, and J. H. Zettl. 1982. International SFTR recording of joint motion and position. In *Amputations, immediate and early prosthetic management,* 240-75. Bern, Stuttgart, Vienna: Hans Huber Publishers.

Hamilton, J. J., and L. K. Ziemer. 1983. Functional anatomy of the human ankle and foot. In *American Academy of Orthopaedic Surgeons. Symposium on the foot and ankle,* 1-14. St. Louis, MO: C. V. Mosby.

International Standards Organizations. 1988. *Basic list of anthropometric measurements.* Draft proposal ISO-DP 7250. Geneva, Switzerland: ISO.

Keegan, J. J. 1953. Alterations of the lumbar curve related to posture and seating. *Journal of Bone and Joint Surgery* 35-A(3).

Letts, M., L. Shapiro, K. Mulder, and O. Klassen. 1984. The windblown hip syndrome in total body cerebral palsy. *Journal of Pediatric Orthopedics* 4:55-62.

Mann, R., N. McCollough III, and S. Sarrafian. 1975. Bio-mechanical analysis system (upper and lower limbs). In *Biomechanical principles and application, atlas of orthotics,* chapters 4, 9, 13, 18. St. Louis, MO: C. V. Mosby.

Medhat, M. A., and J. B. Redford. 1987 (Feb). Prescribed seating systems. In *Physical medicine and rehabilitation: State of the art reviews,* Vol. 1, No. 1, edited by J. B. Redford, 111-36.

Medhat, M. A., and P. Trautman. 1986. Seating devices for the disabled. In *Orthotics etcetera,* edited by J. B. Redford, 654-707. Baltimore: Williams and Wilkins.

National Technical Information Service. 1978. *Anthropometric source book,* Vols. 1, 2, and 3. NASA Report 1024. Springfield.

Norken, L. V. 1983. *Joint structure and functions; A comprehensive analysis.* Philadelphia: F. A. Davis.

Safler, F., S. Bachman, and C. Bazata. 1988. In search of a common language: Uniform terminology for seating and positioning. In *Proceedings of the international conference for the advancement of rehabilitation technology,* 294-95. Washington, DC: RESNA Press.

Scoliosis Research Society. *List of deformities, classifications, and terminology.*

Smith, R., and J. Leslie, eds. 1990. *Rehabilitation engineering.* Boca Raton, FL: CRC Press.

Webster, M. 1976. *Webster's seventh new collegiate dictionary,* 314. Springfield, MA: G&C Merriam Company.

Wells, K. 1968. *Kinesiology.* Philadelphia: W. B. Saunders.

Special Interest Group on Wheeled Mobility and Seating (SIG-09)— Terminology Task Force

Bonnie Boenig, M.Ed., OTR/L
Boenig and Associates Therapy Services, Inc.
173 Front Street
Berea, OH 44017

Clifford Brubaker, Ph.D.
College of Health Related Professions and
  Rehabilitation Sciences
University of Pittsburgh
Pittsburgh, PA 15261

Martin Ferguson-Pell, Ph.D.
Center for Rehabilitation Technology
Helen Hayes Hospital
Route 9W
West Haverstraw, NY 10993

Geoff Fernie, Ph.D., PEng, CCE
West Park Research Rehabilitation Engineering
West Park Hospital
82 Buttonwood Avenue
Toronto, Ontario M6M 2J5

Michael Heinrich
Pin Dot
6001 Gross Point Road
Niles, IL 60648-4027

Doug Hobson, Ph.D.
School of Health & Rehabilitation Science
University of Pittsburgh
915 William Pitt Way
Pittsburgh, PA 15238

Susan Johnson-Taylor, OTR
Shephard Spinal Center
2020 Peachtree Road
Atlanta, GA 30309

Simon Margolis, CO
Rehabilitation Designs, Inc.
1492 Martin Street
Madison, WI 53713

Mohamed A. Medhat, M.D., Ph.D.
Rehabilitation Medicine Services
Saint Joseph Health Center
930 Carondelet Drive, Suite 303
Kansas City, MO 64114

Jean Minkel, PT
Center for Rehabilitation Technology
Helen Hayes Hospital
Route 9W
West Haverstraw, NY 10993

Lynn Monahan, OTR
United Medical
1835 Nonconnah Boulevard, Suite 143
Memphis, TN 38132

Nancy Mulholland, RPT
PO Box 4240
Ventura, CA 93004

Daphne J. Neen
Occupational and Physical Therapy
Sunny Hill Hospital for Children
3644 Slocan Street
Vancouver, British Columbia V5M 3E8

Jessica Presperin, OTR/L, MBA
Rehabilitation Technology Coordinator
Sharp Rehabilitation Hospital
7901 Frost Street
San Diego, CA 92123

Steven Reger, Ph.D.
Musculo Skeletal Research (WB3)
9500 Euclid Avenue
Cleveland, OH 44195-5254

Lori Roxborough, BSR
Sunny Hill Hospital for Children
3544 Slocan Street
Vancouver, British Columbia V5M 3E8

Paul Trautman, CPO
Orthopedic Service Center, Inc.
5341 West 94th Terrace
Mission, KS 66207

Elaine Trefler, OTR, M.Ed.
4215 Yarmouth Dr.
Allison Park, PA 15101

Diane Ward, OTR
543 West Delmont
Chicago, IL 60657

APPENDIX B

. . . .

Technology Overview and Classification*

by D. A. Hobson, Ph.D.

*Reprinted with permission from: Hobson, D. A. 1988. Seating and mobility for the severely disabled. In *Rehabilitation engineering,* edited by J. Leslie, 201-218. Copyright, CRC Press, Inc., Boca Raton, Florida.

Technology Overview and Classification

The rapidly increasing number of commercial options in seating and mobility present many new selection challenges for clinicians and consumers, especially for those first entering the field. No standard system of classification or terminology has been established to facilitate communication among clinicians, students, suppliers, consumers, and researchers.

The classification scheme that follows is an initial attempt and therefore should not be regarded as definitive. This appendix provides a structured frame of reference in terms of highlighting the generic technologies in the field.

The basis of the presentation is a classification system complemented by a descriptive section which identifies and defines the terminology that is in most common use today. Seating technologies will be presented first, followed by mobility technologies.

Seating Technologies— Classification and Terminology

The field of specialized seating is evolving along three distinct tracts, each of which have been guided largely by the needs of distinct user populations. These tracts are: (a) seating for postural control and deformity management (those with cerebral palsy); (b) seating for pressure and postural management (those with spinal cord injuries); and (c) seating for comfort and postural accommodation (those with multiple handicaps and the geriatric population) (figure 4).

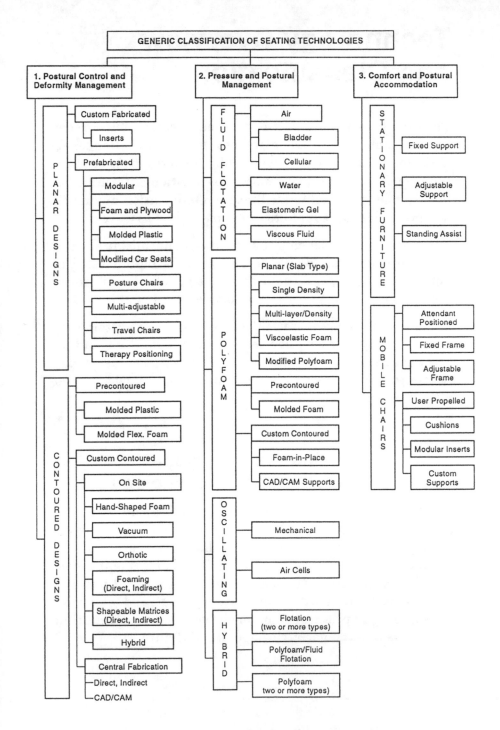

Figure 4. Generic classification of seating technologies.

Postural Control and Deformity
Management Technologies

This area of specialized seating has been guided largely by the needs of children and young adults with cerebral palsy, closed-head injury, or post drowning. Within the cerebral palsy group, the seating needs vary significantly depending on the type and degree of damage to the immature brain. The combination of involuntary muscle activity and deformity results in a diverse array of needs for postural control and support. These needs can range from being only minimal (mildly involved) to being extensive (severely involved).

Seating system designs have evolved in response to these diverse seating needs. The associated technological approaches, as may be seen in the classification scheme in figure 4, have taken two basic directions, those designed with planar (flat) surfaces and those that are contoured to provide more intimate support to the body.

Both main categories can be further subdivided. Planar designs may be either custom fabricated or prefabricated. Contoured designs may be either precontoured or custom contoured. There are various technological approaches that fall within each of these major categories.

Planar Components

Prefabricated. Prefabricated planar seating components are designed with essentially flat surfaces and are produced and sold commercially in stock sizes to meet the size requirements of clients from approximately two years of age to adulthood. Prefabricated planar designs fall into five basic subgroups.

Modular inserts are designed to be inserted into a variety of existing wheelchairs and specialty mobility bases. They are attached to the mobility bases by interfacing hardware which also allows adjustments to critical length, width, and angular positions. Modular inserts are produced in a variety of ways. These are basic foam and plywood construction, molded plastic, and injected molded plastics, such as infant car seats which have been modified to meet special needs.

Posture chairs reflect attempts by the wheelchair industry to meet posturing needs. Posture chairs are essentially standard wheelchair frames to which have been added a variety of planar adjustable pads.

Multi-adjustable systems feature a large number of adjustable planar components with their own integral wheeled bases. They also have a range of complementary accessories such as foot and head supports, trunk supports, and a tray option.

Travel chairs were originally designed to facilitate transportation in the family car. In recent years, the seating arrangements have been refined to include many of the adjustable features found in modular inserts and multi-adjustable systems. However, they remain distinct from the others due to the configuration of the integral wheeled base, designed to allow transport in the front seat of a standard automobile. Travel chairs are generally not suitable for transportation in vans or school buses, unless the company supplies federally approved car seats.

Finally, there are planar prefabricated therapy positioning aids that are commonly used at floor or low level during therapy sessions with younger children (such as corner seats).

Custom-fabricated. Custom-fabricated planar designs are the technology used by most facilities when basic seating inserts are fabricated on site. This is the most direct approach in which vinyl-covered foam is stapled to a plywood substructure (foam and plywood), which in turn is interfaced into a standard wheelchair.

This technology has improved with the advent of commercial interfacing hardware and accessories that readily mount to the planar surfaces (such as headrests and trunk bolsters). Although conceptually simple, the foam-and-plywood approach can become rather complex and labor-intensive when any degree of body fit (custom contouring) is undertaken.

Contoured Components

Increasing the complexity of postural support needs involves the use of seating componentry that increases the area of contact between the body and the seating support (that is, the use of contoured versus planar surfaces).

Two basic technological approaches have been used. The first uses precontoured modules so that the seating components can be manufactured using standard shapes. The second obtains the contours by taking the shape directly from the client. The first approach is termed a precontoured component, and the second is termed a custom-contoured component (figure 4).

Precontoured components. Standardized molds have been designed with symmetrical body shapes and produced in incremental sizes. The molds are then used to reproduce seating support modules using one of several possible industrial manufacturing processes.

Vacuum-formed plastic or molded flexible polyurethane foam are common technologies used to produce the prefabricated modules. Again, adjustable interface hardware is normally used to allow the relative adjustment of the seat and back modules and attachment (interfacing) to standard or integral mobility bases.

The advantage of the prefabricated components is that they are available off the shelf and can be quickly assembled into a functional seating system. This approach is often adequate for those with mild to moderate physical involvement.

However, because the contours are standardized and symmetrical in shape, this approach becomes inappropriate when intimately fitting body support is needed, as is usually the case when deformity necessitates custom-contoured seat and back modules.

Custom contoured. When custom-contoured components are required, one of two basic directions may be taken. One may choose a design that allows complete on-site fabrication and fitting of the system or an approach that uses a central fabrication facility as part of the fabrication process.

ON-SITE FABRICATION TECHNIQUES

There are five distinct technical approaches that are now used to construct custom-contoured seating components on site, or within the immediate locale in which the seating services are provided (figure 4). The main differences in these approaches are a result of the generic technology employed, the technical skills required, the fabrication time, the intimacy of the resulting fit, and the aesthetics of the final product.

- Hand-shaped foam—This approach is usually considered the most basic or original of the technologies used to obtain custom-contoured components. The seating modules are hand-carved in a trial-and-error process from a block of higher-density foam to fit the contours of the body.

  These blocks may then be covered with vinyl to provide an outer surface that is both durable and moisture-proof. This basic approach is usually labor-intensive and requires considerable technical skill to obtain an intimate fit, especially when accommodation of gross deformities is necessary.

- Vacuum consolidation—The vacuum consolidation technique is a more common approach and is used in several ways. The basic technique consists of using a flexible, airtight membrane filled with particles, such as polystyrene beads or plastic injection molding pellets. Once the flexible membrane is shaped around the body part (pelvis or trunk, or both), evacuation of the air causes the shape to become rigid.

  If a glue has been mixed in with the particles prior to shaping, then the resulting shape can be used to fabricate the definitive seating system on site. This is termed the direct vacuum consolidation technique.

  If the airtight bag and particles are used without glue, the vacuum consolidation shape can be reused to obtain a negative impression of the body shape.

This negative impression is then used to make a positive plaster impression, which in turn is used to make the definitive seating components using either a modified orthotic approach or a central fabrication approach.

When vacuum consolidation is used as the means for transferring shape (that is, negative to positive impression), it is termed the indirect approach.

- Modified orthotic approach—A traditional orthotic approach has been used for many years to make spinal support orthoses, foot/ankle orthoses, and so on. A negative impression of the body segment is obtained using plaster bandage. A positive plaster mold is made by filling up the negative cavity with plaster. The plaster positive is modified to obtain the degree of correction or support required by the final orthosis. High-temperature, vacuum-formable plastic (such as polypropylene) is formed over the plaster positive to make the final appliance.

In the modified orthotic approach, as often used in specialized seating, the vacuum consolidation technique is used to obtain the negative impression and the plaster mold. The plaster mold includes both the pelvis and trunk, which results in a one-piece plastic seating support. Interfacing into the wheelchair and addition of chest and pelvic restraints and head and foot supports completes the modified orthotic seating system.

The orthotic technique usually requires high technical skill and considerable technical time. It is not an approach recommended for those who lack conventional orthotic training or experiences. However, this approach probably results in the most intimate body fit of all the seating technologies in use today.

Problems can arise with one-piece, intimately fitting supports when seat-to-back angles require changing, or when frequent modifications are necessary due to rapid growth.

- Foaming—Polyurethane foams are usually manufactured from two chemically reacting components, one an isocyanate and the other a resin, both liquid at room temperature. When these components are mixed in the correct proportions, a chemical reaction generates an innocuous blowing agent (carbon dioxide) that causes the foam to rise and form cells, thereby increasing its volume 15 to 20 times.

This polymerization and expansion process can be used to obtain custom-contoured shapes of body supports. If the foaming process uses the person directly as the mold, it is termed a foam-in-place or direct foaming process. If the foaming is done against a plaster positive or a mold of the body, it is termed a foam-in-box or indirect process.

Polyurethane foams may be formulated to be either flexible or rigid upon polymerization. Flexible foams are used in furniture cushions as well as many traditional wheelchair cushions. Rigid foams have been most commonly used for spray-on industrial insulations.

The unpolymerized isocyanate component can be harmful if exposed to skin, eyes, or mucous membranes, especially for those with respiratory hypersensitivity. Therefore, it is very important that the isocyanate component be of the MDI and not the TDI variety, since the MDI type is much less hazardous.

Rather extensive toxicity studies have been done to evaluate the level of risk to clients during the foam-in-place process (Hobson and Tooms 1981). One study, in addition to pointing out the fact that no problems have been reported after over 500 clinical applications, suggests that the risk to health of both clients and staff is minimal. However, the industry's handling precautions must be observed.

Applications with people who have cerebral palsy have been mainly those with severe discomfort problems due to deformity. The main applications have been for those with spinal cord injury and Duchenne muscular dystrophy who are seeking comfort through resilient support.

Although the two-piece, foam-in-place system can be used to quickly produce (within three to four hours) custom-contoured resilient seat and back modules, successful polymerization of flexible foams does require precise mixing and handling techniques. Also, the desired body posture must be correct or the process will have to be repeated.

The indirect foaming process will be described further under the discussion on central fabrication.

• Shapeable matrices—Another technical approach that bypasses the positive plaster step in producing a custom-contoured seating system is the use of shapeable matrices.

Injection-molded interlocking plastic components are assembled into a flexible, one-piece mat that can be shaped to the contours of the body. Once shaped, friction-locking nodes are tightened and the shape is fixed. Spaces between the plastic components allow inspection for fit and permit air circulation even after a slip-on cover has been added.

The initial design called for direct application and shaping to the body using an adjustable fitting frame (Cousins et al. 1983). However, clinical use with more involved individuals has necessitated the use of a positive model obtained by using the vacuum consolidation technique. This indirect shapeable matrix method allows completion of the system on the workbench, without having to keep the client suspended in the fitting frame for long periods of time.

Experience with over 100 fittings in the United States has shown this method to be a very labor-intensive approach. Very few facilities have been able to complete a shapeable matrix system in less than two days, especially when severe deformities are present.

Loosening of the friction nodes has been experienced, which causes inadvertent loss of shape or loss of parts. The one-piece matrix construction and its tubular support structure have proven difficult to modify as necessitated by growth or postural changes.

Thus, it is recommended that the shapeable matrix approach be reserved for the most difficult applications in which total body support is a necessity. Initial component cost, the fabrication labor, plus repair and follow-up make the matrix one of the most expensive seating approaches. It is recommended for use only by those who have had extensive training given by instructors who have had at least 50 fitting experiences.

- Hybrid—The hybrid custom-contoured category is added as a reminder that, in reality, seating solutions often require the application of more than one of the above technologies in order to meet the unique needs of an individual. In fact, seating systems often combine various technologies, particularly for severely disabled individuals.

In difficult cases, it can be necessary to exploit the advantages of several technical approaches. For example, a planar plywood, foam, and vinyl seat may be combined with a contoured vacuum-consolidated back (Bead System). This approach may facilitate transfers from the wheelchair but allows the necessary control for the trunk.

In other cases, a custom-contoured seat may be required in order to maintain pelvic and lower limb control, whereas planar components would be adequate for support of the trunk.

CENTRAL FABRICATION

- Direct/Indirect—As previously discussed, vacuum consolidation and foam-in-place technologies provide methods for efficiently obtaining negative shapes (impressions) of body shapes.

In the vacuum consolidation approach, flexible, air-tight bags or the stretchy surface of an airtight fitting frame is formed around the person who has been positioned in an appropriate seated posture. The pelvic area is usually formed first, followed by the trunk.

Evacuation of the air from around the particles causes the mechanical interlocking and retention of the negative shape after the person is removed from the molding frame. Plaster bandage is then used to recover or reproduce the negative shape of the body part from the vacuum consolidation bag (indirect method).

Once reference marks and appropriate documentation are added, the positive shape(s) can be sent to a central location for reproduction of the shape(s) into molded flexible foam seating components.

The foam modules are completely finished and placed in an adjustable interfacing frame by the central facility. The seating system is then returned to the clinic site, complete with the ordered accessories, ready for final fitting. The flexible foam modules are produced by the central fabricator using the indirect (foam-in-box) foaming technique.

A variation of the above central fabrication process uses the direct foaming technique to obtain the shapes. In this case, rigid urethane polymers are mixed and injected into a plastic bag against which the client has been positioned. The foam rises and forces the flexible bag around the seated subject. The foam sets quickly and retains the seated shape.

The rigid modules are then sent directly to a central fabrication facility, where they are trimmed, padded, covered, and assembled into an adjustable interface. The interfaced modules, complete with accessories, can then be returned to the clinical site for final fitting.

This latter approach bypasses the need to transfer the shape from the vacuum consolidation bag using the plaster bandage, as in the previous indirect approach. The disadvantage is that, with the direct foaming approach, the person must be positioned correctly before the foaming begins; otherwise, the process will need to be repeated if significant positioning errors have been made.

In addition, it is possible to obtain planar custom-fabricated components from several fabrication facilities. This approach necessitates sending in fairly detailed dimensions on standardized measurement forms. The foam and plywood components are then fabricated to specifications and returned to the fitting site ready for interfacing with the wheeled base and final fitting.

This approach can be an alternative if very limited technical resources exist on site. The limitation is that it becomes difficult to communicate body measurements accurately, especially if asymmetrical deformity exists. As a result, it is suggested that any centralized, custom-fabricated approach that relies on communication by linear body measurements be limited to clients with only mild to moderate physical involvement.

- CAD/CAM—Industrial technology routinely uses computerized equipment as a means of recording or designing shapes of complex objects. The shapes are stored in the computer as digital information, a process termed *computer-aided design* (CAD). The design of automobile body shapes is an example of this technology.

A companion technology, termed *computer-aided manufacturing* (CAM), uses the stored digital information to control the operation of manufacturing equipment. Numerically or digitally controlled (NCR) machines can quickly reproduce the shapes derived by the CAD procedure. The process can also be programmed to modify the digital information (shapes) so that the final shapes can be changed to meet specified requirements.

Current research (Krouskop et al. 1987) and clinical trials have demonstrated the technical feasibility of acquiring body segment shapes and then reproducing these shapes with numerically controlled shaping equipment. The shapes are usually cut from blocks of flexible or rigid foam.

The CAD/CAM-produced modules could be the custom-contoured postural supports used in seating systems. However, as with other seating approaches, the modules still must be covered to provide the desired durability and aesthetics and then interfaced into a mobility base.

The CAD/CAM approach is indeed complex. However, if efficient, low-cost CAD devices can be developed for rapidly acquiring the body shapes in clinical settings, the approach has significant commercial promise.

The main advantage is that, because the product of the CAD technique is stored digital information (which in this case defines the body segment shape), it can be transmitted electronically to a central CAM site for rapid production of the support modules.

Also, once a person's shape is obtained, this information can easily be stored or modified for use in subsequent replacements. Combined data from many sources could be used to generate standard shapes for production of prefabricated contoured modules. Selection of the standard module could then be made based on only a few critical dimensions.

CAD/CAM technology is only in its infancy in customized seating fabrication. Although technically appealing, it should be remembered that it is only a technique for streamlining the central fabrication process. All the other steps of evaluation—interfacing with wheeled bases, adding accessories, and so forth—must still be done.

Pressure and Posture Management Technologies

Individuals with spinal cord injury are at risk of developing pressure sores in the tissues overlying the pelvic area. Many types of wheelchair cushions have been developed in an attempt to control pressure over the bony prominences of the pelvis (figure 4).

Dissipation of body heat to prevent moisture buildup and maintenance of postural stability are also important factors that have influenced cushion design. A wide range of materials, geometric configurations, and mechanical technologies have been tested and used in cushion designs. Clinical experience clearly indicates that the requirements of individuals vary widely and that no single design meets every need (Garber and Krouskop 1984).

The development of seating technologies designed for pressure and postural management has followed an evolutionary path somewhat different from technology designed for people with cerebral palsy (postural control and deformity management).

In general, cushion designs for the population with spinal cord injury are first categorized by the media or mechanical technique used to obtain the pressure relief, rather than on whether the surface profile is planar or contoured. As indicated in figure 4, the basic media approaches are fluid flotation, polyfoams, and oscillating devices. A fourth subcategory, hybrids, provides a means of classifying designs that use two or more of the first three approaches.

Fluid Flotation

Four fluid mediums have been used in cushion designs: air, water, viscous fluid, and elastomer gels.

Air-filled designs have taken several directions. Two of the most common approaches are: (a) configured bladders or rubber membrane designs, and (b) a cellular approach.

The most common cellular cushion has a large number of individual balloons (cells). This approach tends to minimize any hammocking effect as well as permit air movement through the support structure. It is important in any air-filled design that the appropriate air pressure be maintained. Overinflation or inadvertent loss of support pressure is possibly the most serious drawback to the air-type flotation devices.

Water-filled cushions are less common. Although they provide good dissipation of body heat, leaks and excessive weight are noted problem areas. Again, the hammocking effect created by the covering membrane can negate the pressure equalization attributes of fluid suspension.

Elastomeric gels can be considered a very high viscous fluid, since gel does exhibit flow and pressure distribution properties similar to a fluid. Gel cushions are produced from materials such as silicone elastomers, chosen to have a viscosity or consistency similar to body fat.

Gel cushions also provide good heat dissipation but are usually heavy, and gel leakage has been a problem with some designs. Pressure distribution characteristics can be affected greatly by the design of the confining membrane and its outer covering material(s).

More recently, high viscosity fluids contained in oversized flexible membranes are being used. The high viscous fluid exhibits pressure equalization properties of a fluid but is free to flow within the confines of the membrane from areas of highest loading. This, in effect, creates a custom-contouring effect. This approach is now used in several commercial applications.

Polyfoam Designs

Polyurethane foams (and some latex-based varieties) have been the mainstay of cushion technology over the years, particularly for those individuals at low to moderate pressure sore risk. The pressure relief characteristics of foam cushions depend on the inherent mechanical properties of the foam, whether it is used in a single or multilayered "slab" configuration or contoured to the pelvic area, either through precontoured molding or custom contouring to the precise shape of a person's pelvic area.

Planar (slab type). In general, planar foam cushions are the most versatile because bilayering with different densities, altering geometry through cutouts, and finishing with suitable slip-on covers can be accomplished with minimal technical support and resulting cost. Cushion thickness can be altered easily and the inherent light weight and simplicity of wheelchair insertion facilitates transfers.

Disadvantages are that their life is relatively short (6 to 12 months), and most cushions cannot be washed readily without reducing their effectiveness (Noble et al. 1984). Also, the pressure-relieving characteristics may not be adequate without significant modifications, especially for those in the moderate to high risk group.

Planar polyfoam cushions are designed with many foam types and configurations. Slabs of foam up to 4″ thick may be used in a single-density design. Foams of varying thicknesses, types, and densities may be combined to gain the advantages of each type in a multilayer/density design (Ferguson-Pell et al. 1986).

A variation of the conventional polyurethane foam technology is to introduce a viscous fluid into the cellular foam structure. This combination creates viscoelastic properties which exhibit characteristics of both the standard polyfoam and viscous fluid flotation devices.

Although the pressure distribution capabilities are enhanced, viscoelastic cushions are influenced significantly by ambient temperatures. Shock absorption and postural stability characteristics are usually superior to traditional polyfoams.

It is important to realize that, in clinical practice, a great deal of creative design is undertaken in terms of modifying planar (slab type) foams. The geometry of the slab is modified through ischial area "cutouts," "egg crating" by the manufacturer, or cutting serrations in one or both surfaces to enhance pressure distribution or other mechanical properties of the foam.

The art and science of modifying polyfoams has been addressed by several researchers (Ferguson-Pell et al. 1980; Ferguson-Pell et al. 1986; Garber and Krouskop 1984; Garber, Krouskop, and Carter 1978; Krouskop et al. 1983).

Precontoured polyfoam. More recently, designers have attempted to distribute pressure away from bony prominences through the design of precontoured support surfaces.

Precontoured designs provide an opportunity to reduce pressures in the genital area, thus reducing the likelihood of constriction to the urethra. Also, increased air circulation can help to reduce humidity buildup. Tissue loading is moved away from the ischial prominences to surrounding gluteal tissues. However, this tends to create a "rim effect" of high pressures.

The prefabricated contoured cushions are made by injecting polyurethane foam into standard molds. A dip or spray-on covering material increases the durability of the cushion and reduces moisture penetration. The developers of Vaso-Para, one example of this technology, have published information on the rationale for the shape used and the results of their clinical trials (Perkash et al. 1984).

Figure 5 illustrates a number of the more common commercial cushion technologies discussed above.

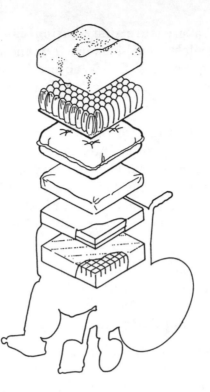

Figure 5. Examples of technologies used in pressure and posture management. *(Courtesy of Rehabilitation Press)*

Custom Contoured

Foam-in-place. Contouring of polyfoam to meet the shape of an individual has the promise of reducing the shear stresses inherent in slab foam designs. Design of the support surfaces can be readily individualized to redistribute pressure similar to the precontoured approach.

CAD/CAM. As indicated previously, CAD/CAM technology has been used to produce seat cushions for individuals with spinal cord injuries on an experimental basis (Brubaker 1988) and more recently for clinical trials.

The promise of designing and producing support surfaces to meet individualized pressure redistribution needs offers exciting possibilities for this computerized approach. The availability of clinical tools that can rapidly record body shapes will most likely dictate the feasibility and degree of acceptance of the CAD/CAM approach.

Oscillating Devices

Early research showed the relationship between pressure and time as it relates to the formation of pressure sores (Kosiak 1959; Rodgers 1974). Relatively high pressures could be tolerated by pelvic tissues if the duration was kept short. Lower pressures were necessary if the weight-bearing time was increased.

This basic relationship, combined with subsequent studies and clinical experiences, forms the basis for the clinical guidelines used today in establishing acceptable pressure levels and decompression (pressure-relieving) frequencies.

The cushion designs discussed above are either static or quasi-dynamic devices in which periodic changes of body position are required to assure sufficient reduction in pressure levels through weight relief of supporting tissues. These static designs all attempt to equalize or redistribute pressure over the contact surface of the pelvis. That is, they attempt to minimize the pressures acting on susceptible areas of the pelvis (the ischial tuberosities).

Oscillating designs alter the pelvic pressure profile independent of the user. In general, they adhere to the principle that locally high pressures can be tolerated provided the duration is kept within prescribed limits. Several approaches have been pursued, one basically a mechanical design, and the other undulating air cells on bellows.

One experimental wheelchair seat consisted of a series of rollers on a chain drive that moved under the person at a predetermined speed (Kosiak 1976). Although the time/pressure profiles were within tolerable limits described in a previous work (Kosiak 1959), the complexity, cost, and bulk of the device has precluded its commercialization and clinical use.

Talley Medical, Ltd., of England, has produced oscillating air cell devices. The first, termed the Ripple Seat, consists of eight adjacently mounted air tubes (each measuring 2″ by 14″). Alternate air tubes are connected to a common air manifold which, in turn, is connected to a small battery-powered, portable oscillating pump. Each series of four air tubes is inflated as the other series of four tubes is being deflated. The effect is an oscillating system which produces intermittent high pressure followed by low pressure to alternate areas of the pelvic surface.

A more recent design, termed the Air Bellows Support, uses a matrix of cellular air bellows (3″ high by 1½″ diameter) connected to a similar manifold/oscillating air pump. The pump is designed to allow adjustment of the pressure levels and the frequency of pressure changes across the bellows matrix. A warning device alerts users to system failures so that corrective action can be taken.

Clinical experiences with any of the oscillating devices in North America is very limited. The approach is technically intriguing and may offer significant advances in pressure management in the years ahead.

Hybrid Systems

As with the technology used in postural control and deformity management, pressure management technologies do not all fit neatly into the above classification scheme. The Hybrid category permits the classification of cushion designs that employ two or more of the above approaches.

For example, several of the fluid flotation mediums have been combined into a single cushion design. Others use water within an air bladder. In another approach, elastomeric gels and related high viscous fluids have been combined with polyfoam structures. For example, the Jay cushion uses a precontoured polyfoam substructure with a top surface membrane filled with a high viscosity fluid, whereas the Akros-Zero Pressure uses a precontoured plastic substructure with a gel-impregnated polyfoam top layer.

Ferguson-Pell et al. (1986) succinctly describe the key factors involved in designing multimedia/layered modular cushions to address the specific needs of individuals with spinal cord injury. A review of this work is recommended to anyone contemplating design or development of hybrid-type cushions for the management of pressure sores.

A glaring omission from the generic classification scheme are technologies and devices that specifically address the posturing needs of individuals with spinal cord injury. Observation of individuals five years or more post-injury suggests that spinal and pelvic deformities due to inappropriate sitting posture are a common outcome among this population (Hobson and Nwaobi 1985; Zackarkow 1984).

The posturing tools developed and experiences gained with those who have cerebral palsy are slowly filtering over to the population with spinal cord injuries. Hopefully, future research and clinical practice will take a more holistic approach to seating of those with spinal cord injuries, and not remain overwhelmed by the immensity of the pressure management problem.

Comfort and Postural Accommodation

Although elderly persons account for the largest number of wheelchair users (Bardsley 1984), seating technologies for the elderly population are still in their infancy. For example, relatively few commercial products have been developed specifically to enhance the care or independent functioning of older people in nursing homes. Even fewer attempts have been made to develop systems that facilitate the maintenance of these groups in the home and community.

The existing designs and technologies employed can be classified into broad subgroups which are based largely on the manner in which the devices are intended to be used, that is, whether the device is intended to be stationary sitting furniture or mobile, or whether it is to be propelled by an attendant or by the user.

Stationary Furniture

Several manufacturers offer chairs which attempt to address the special needs of elderly persons. Comfort, as it is with the general population, is the main design objective because of the many hours per day older people spend sitting. Several researchers have done work in this area of seating comfort by exploring seat and back contours (Bardsley 1984; Fernie, Holden, and Lanau 1987). Most current stationary chairs, whether they be residential recliner models or nursing home bedside chairs, are designed to facilitate sitting down and standing up.

Mobile Chairs

Many older persons who have problems walking become dependent on a conventional wheelchair for mobility. For many, the wheelchair—never designed for long-term sitting—is their primary chair. A recent study of nursing home residents indicated that the standard wheelchair is uncomfortable for 47% of those who sit for four or more hours per day (Shaw 1988).

Commercial wheelchair cushions have been used in an attempt to improve sitting comfort. In addition to conventional wheelchairs, some elderly persons, especially those in nursing homes, use upholstered chairs, referred to as stroke or geriatric chairs. With few exceptions, these chairs are equipped with small wheels and require an attendant to move them from one place to another. The original nonreclining geriatric chairs, sometimes referred to as feeding chairs, offer little user comfort.

The reclining stroke chairs are essentially recliner chairs on wheels and are considered more comfortable than conventional wheelchairs by nursing home residents. Recent research and development efforts have resulted in chairs offering improved comfort and convenience (Bardsley 1984; Fernie, Holden, and Lanau 1987). Many elderly persons who require this type of chair are small women and/or those who have deformities. These newer designs offer customizing for size and postural support.

Mobility Technologies— Classification and Terminology

In general, personal mobility technologies have developed along two parallel paths: designs intended to be manually propelled and those designed to use external battery power as the propulsion energy source (figure 6).

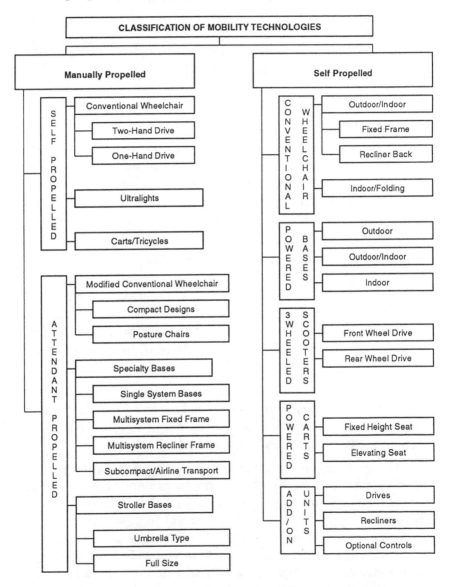

Figure 6. General classification of mobility technologies.

In the manually propelled group, two large subcategories emerge: those devices designed to be propelled primarily by the user (self-propelled) and those designed to be attendant-propelled.

Manually Propelled
· ·

Self-Propelled

In the marketplace today there are three distinctive design approaches inherent in self-propelled mobility devices: (1) the conventional folding wheelchair and its close derivatives, (2) ultralight or lightweight wheelchairs, and (3) carts and tricycles.

Conventional wheelchair. As previously mentioned, Everest and Jennings are credited with developing and marketing the conventional steel tube X-frame wheelchair which has been the standard of the industry since the late 1930s. Of course, varieties of both the three- and four-wheeled designs existed prior to that time.

The conventional X-frame wheelchair is now produced in hundreds of different models around the world. When all the possible optional accessories (such as wheel sizes/types, armrest styles, footrest/legrest styles, upholstery width/height/ colors, and so forth) are added to the large number of basic models, the permutations of possible configurations extend into the thousands.

The basic conventional folding wheelchair is designed with two large rear wheels which are used for self-propulsion with two hands. The front wheels are castered to allow high maneuverability and steering from the rear wheels.

This basic design is a very effective means of mobility, particularly on indoor surfaces. Efforts to replace the dual rear wheel propulsion/steering system with levers or crank devices have had very limited commercial success, particularly in North America. However, for those cases in which only one arm is functionally able to provide the propulsion energy, single-drive wheel or one-handed wheelchairs have been developed.

More recently, single-lever drive versions have gained clinical acceptance. A primarily European variation of the conventional wheelchair configuration mounts the large drive wheels in the front and the castered wheels in the rear.

Most insert-type seating systems (that is, those that do not have integral bases) have been developed to allow rapid attachment to and detachment from conventional wheelchairs. This has been possible since the majority of the X-frame designs have two parallel seat tubes (rails) and two parallel back tubes (uprights) to which the standard sling-type upholstery is attached.

This basic configuration has permitted the design of standard interfaces (attachment hardware) so that modular seating inserts can be used in a large number of different conventional wheelchairs.

This basic configuration comprises possibly 40% to 50% of the modular seating done today in North America. Another 40% uses posture chairs, travel chairs, or multi-adjustable commercial systems, such as the Mulholland Growth Guidance System. In the latter case, a wheelchair is not required. The remaining 20% uses mobility configurations from one of the categories below.

Ultralights or lightweight wheelchairs. The quest for enhanced mobility, especially related to recreation and athletic pursuits, has fostered the design and development of a new generation of wheelchairs—the high-performance chairs known as ultralights or lightweight wheelchairs (figure 7).

Many of the ultralight designs have taken a significant departure from the conventional X-frame wheelchair. The use of high-strength, low-weight materials, alternate base and seat configurations, improved wheel designs, and drastically enhanced aesthetics have all been combined to evolve this new "breed" of self-propelled mobility devices.

The leaders in innovation have primarily been small, new companies which targeted a marketplace that was seeking mobility alternatives. Active persons with paraplegia who

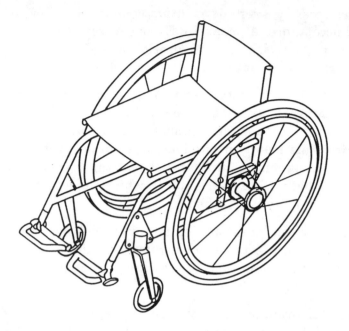

Figure 7. Contemporary ultralight design showing adjustments which alter body center of gravity location relative to the drive wheels. Tracking adjustments of both casters and drive wheels are also possible in many models. Frame designs may be either folding or rigid. Seats and backs provide more firm (flat) support in contrast to traditional sling-type upholstery. *(Courtesy of Rehabilitation Press).*

were involved in athletics were the dominant early users. Today, many active people are using ultralight designs, even very young children.

The ultralight evolution has created a special challenge when alternate seating arrangements are required. In general, ultralight wheelchairs provide even less body support than the conventional sling-type wheelchair.

Ultralight designs have not adopted a standard seat frame configuration; therefore the interfacing of standard seating modules into the many commercial varieties has presented an interesting design challenge. Efforts are now underway to develop interfacing hardware that will allow use of existing and future seating technologies in ultralight bases.

Carts/tricycles. The importance of encouraging independent mobility at an early age has been recognized for several years (Trefler and Marcrum 1987). In response to this need, several carts and modified tricycles have been developed.

The concept is to allow the nonambulatory child who has sufficient limb function (for instance, with spina bifida or mild to moderate cerebral palsy) to be independently mobile. The child with spina bifida, for example, is encouraged to transfer independently from the floor to a low-level cart.

Other designs offer hand-crank propulsion. There are also a number of modified tricycles that can be used by children who have varying degrees of limb function and control.

The devices usually have trunk supports and ways of fixing the feet to the pedals. Some models use hand cranks combined with foot pedals to facilitate reciprocal motion.

Of equal importance are the high performance "trikes" used by active adults for recreational activities. Many new designs, discussed further in a later section, are becoming available.

Attendant-Propelled

The second major group of manually propelled mobility devices are those designed to be propelled by an attendant or caregiver. These designs may be classified in three groups: modified conventional wheelchairs, specialty bases, and stroller bases (figure 6).

Modified conventional wheelchairs. In response to those who cannot propel a conventional (large drive wheel) wheelchair or need additional body support, the industry has produced modified conventional wheelchairs to address a variety of special needs.

Most designs are basically the conventional X-frame wheelchair which has been modified in several ways. For example, if the large drive wheels are removed and replaced with smaller wheels (8" to 12" in diameter), these chairs become more compact, lighter weight, and are commonly used as airport or hospital transport chairs. They usually fold to smaller sizes and therefore allow for easier stowage in car trunks.

A second group of modified conventional wheelchairs intended primarily for attendant propulsion are the posture chairs. This type has varying amounts of seating adaptations added to the frame of a conventional wheelchair. Headrests, trunk bolsters, adjustable abduction blocks, and adjustable planar or contoured seating and back modules are common features.

Most designs retain the large rear wheels which also permit user propulsion on hard surfaces if the prerequisite upper limb function is present. However, most individuals who require additional postural support lack the necessary ability to propel these rather heavy and cumbersome designs. In most cases, the seating arrangements do not readily remove from the chair, making folding for transport and stowage difficult.

Specialty bases. The term "specialty bases" has been reserved for those attendant-propelled bases designed specifically to meet specialized seating/mobility requirements.

Some bases are designed as part of a proprietary seating system and therefore are termed single-system bases. Other bases have been designed to accept a variety of seating systems and are therefore termed multisystem bases. In general, differences in the multisystem bases are based on the seating frame design. Some have a fixed frame and others have a built-in recliner frame feature.

The final subgroup consists of the subcompact transport chairs. These are mobility bases, of considerable design sophistication, that can be collapsed into a small volume. These are used in applications such as on-board aircraft transport where the chair must be narrow enough to negotiate aircraft aisles and then be collapsed for on-board stowage. Varying degrees of body support are available to assure user comfort and security during the transport process.

Stroller bases. Stroller bases have played an important role in mobility of people with physical disabilities. They are lightweight, compact, and a readily acceptable means of transporting children in the community. In response to the special needs of persons with disabilities, the industry has produced modified stroller designs that will transport individuals as heavy as 200 pounds.

Basically, strollers fall within two categories: those with an umbrella-type folding design with flexible sling seats, and those with firm seats which are usually full-sized and less compact when folded.

The postures imposed by the sling seats are usually not appropriate for all-day use. Therefore seating inserts are often added in place of the sling seats if individuals are to be seated in the stroller bases for long periods of time.

Carefully designed interfacing allows easy removal so that the compact folding feature is retained. The full-sized version usually has a firm seat and back, a posturing improvement over the sling-type supports. However, lateral trunk supports and pelvic blocks are usually not available in these full-sized designs.

Caution is called for when considering strollers as the primary base to use with seating applications. It must be remembered that stroller bases have not been designed for use as transportation bases in school buses or vans. Generally any tie-down apparatus is not appropriate, since the frames of the stroller bases are not designed to withstand the crash loads that would be imposed by even the smallest impact.

Battery-Powered Bases

The second mobility category (figure 6) encompasses battery-powered devices. This group can be subdivided into five distinguishable subgroups: a) conventional wheelchairs, b) powered bases, c) three-wheeled scooters, d) powered carts, and e) add-on units.

Conventional Powered Wheelchairs

The conventional X-frame wheelchair, modified to include batteries, motors, and controllers, has been the standard of the industry since 1957. As in the case of the manually propelled models, the permutations of optional models and accessories is extensive.

Over the years the primary innovations have included increased power (12 to 24 volts), quieter and more efficient motors, and increased control options, permitting the tailoring of controller responses to the varying needs of users. Newly designed drive wheels, frames, caster wheels, and improved overall aesthetics have also been achieved in recent years.

Since the basic design has evolved around the X-frame, belt-driven design, its best performance has been limited to hard, smooth, outdoor terrain or indoor environments (outdoor/indoor). Most versions have a fixed frame; however, models with reclining back options are also available. Modified vans or buses are the most practical way of transporting conventional powered wheelchairs on a daily basis.

A second subgroup based on the conventional design is intended primarily for indoor use. These wheelchairs feature lighter motors, smaller and lightweight drive wheels, smaller energy sources (12 volts), and removable components to facilitate folding for transport. The compromise is that negotiation of outdoor terrain, especially steep slopes or long distances, is limited.

Powered Bases

More recent innovations in battery-powered mobility are powered bases. The new bases are robust in design and have large, powerful, direct-drive power trains coupled to smaller diameter and wider gauged drive wheels.

The front caster wheels are also more robust, larger in diameter, and wider gauged, thereby rendering much better overall outdoor performance. Smaller diameter wheels allow a narrower overall chair width while still maintaining large ground contact area under the wheels.

The basic concept of this design is to accept multiple types of seating arrangements, from the conventional sling-type seat to the plush office designs. If necessary, the seating width can be wider than the wheelbase, since the seat does not need to fit between the large drive wheels, as in the case of the conventional powered wheelchair. This effectively reduces the width of the overall unit, especially when larger seating options are needed.

Some designs will allow disassembly into component parts in the event that car transport is essential. However, this is not usually practical as a daily routine.

Powered bases are designed to be used in three basic ways. There are those that have large, powerful drive trains with large on-board energy sources that provide superior outdoor performance, especially when high speed at longer distances is necessary.

Other powered bases are designed to be competitive in the outdoor/indoor market previously dominated by the conventional powered wheelchair. As indicated earlier, the newer powered bases offer improved outdoor performance without sacrifice of indoor maneuverability when compared to the conventional wheelchair designed for outdoor/indoor use. Several models have been designed primarily for indoor use.

In general, powered bases have captured a significant portion of the market. All major manufacturers are now producing powered base models. Several are offering accessories such as powered full-bodied reclining frames and innovative control options.

The new controllers can facilitate integration with other technologies, such as environmental control devices, communication aids, and access to computer workstations. Powered base innovations are to powered mobility as ultralights have been to manually propelled mobility.

Three-Wheeled Scooters

Three-wheeled scooters offer an alternative form of powered mobility for adults who may not require the additional features offered by conventional powered wheelchairs or powered bases.

Powered scooters have been designed primarily for use in indoor environments. They are designed with two small rear wheels and a single front wheel (figure 8). Steering is most commonly done by tiller control of the front wheel.

Seats on these scooters are usually bucket type mounted on a central pedestal. Seat height can be readily adjusted, and a swivel action facilitates entry or egress from the seat. Postural control or pressure management is usually not a consideration with this type of device.

The initial designs were front-wheel drives in that the drive motor was contained in the hub of the front wheel. Later designs have featured a rear-drive configuration in that the two rear wheels are power driven and the front is used for steering only.

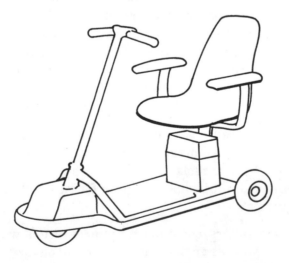

Figure 8. A typical scooter design. *(Courtesy of Rehabilitation Press)*

In general, scooters are used mainly indoors by people who can ambulate for short distances but require powered mobility to transverse longer distances. Shopping malls, schools, amusement parks, hospitals, or buildings with long corridors are ideal sites for scooter use. In general, scooters are less expensive than conventional wheelchairs or powered bases.

Powered Carts

As in the case of manual mobility, powered carts are being used to give young children opportunities to explore their environment. One group of designs is similar to three-wheel, rear-drive scooters but has fixed-height seats low to the floor to facilitate transfer and safety.

Powered cars have been used by children as young as 18 months who lack the ability to propel manually but who have the functional ability to operate a joystick or some alternate control device.

A variation to the fixed-seat-height cart are those with elevating seats which can allow young persons to be at floor level and then elevate themselves to a seated height commensurate with changing activities. Some also allow the attachment of a standing frame to allow mobility in the standing posture.

It is exciting to witness powered vehicles being designed and marketed for young people who have no other means of independent mobility.

Add-on Power Units

A powered accessories industry has paralleled the powered wheelchair industry for many years. These powered options include drive units, recliners, and optional controllers. For example, there are power drive units that can be clamped to manually propelled wheelchairs that can well serve the needs of persons requiring only limited or temporary powered mobility.

Other power accessories that can be added to manually powered chairs are powered recliners and/or powered tilt-in-space features. With activation of a simple on/off switch, recliners can recline the back rest only or tilt a full body frame which changes the total body orientation in space.

Some of the back recline units are rather sophisticated in design in that they have moving seat and/or back modules to minimize the relative movement between the person and the reclining seat component(s). These designs are valuable contributions for those who require powered postural adjustments in order to enhance function or independently seek relief from pressure or discomfort.

Several small companies have specialized in producing optional control devices that either replace or supplement the controller provided by the original equipment manufacturer. These devices provide control options using the chin, head, voice, limited hand motion, and so on. They can also provide access to other devices, such as communication aids, computers, and environmental control devices.

References

Bardsley, G. I. 1984. The Dundee seating programme. *Physiotherapy* 70:59.

Brubaker, C. E. 1988. Personal communication.

Cousins, S. J., K. E. Ackerley, K. N. Jones, and T. R. T. Rodwell. 1983. *Matrix body system. Report.* London: Department of Mechanical Engineering, Bioengineering Centre, Roehampton.

Ferguson-Pell, M., G. V. B. Cochran, V. R. Palmieri, and J. B. Brunski. 1986. Development of a modular wheelchair cushion for spinal cord injured persons. *Journal of Rehabilitation Research and Development* 23:63.

Ferguson-Pell, M. W., J. C. Wilkie, J. B. Reswick, and J. C. Barbenel. 1980. Pressure sore prevention for the wheelchair-bound spinal injury patient. *Paraplegia* 18:42-51.

Fernie, G. R., J. M. Holden, and K. Lanau. 1987. Chair design for the elderly. In *Proceedings, third international seating symposium*, 212-218. Washington, DC: RESNA Press.

Garber, S. L., and T. A. Krouskop. 1984. Wheelchair cushion modification and its effect on pressure. *Archives of Physical Medicine and Rehabilitation* 65:579.

Garber, S. L., T. A. Krouskop, and R. E. Carter. 1978. A system for clinically evaluating wheelchair pressure relief cushions. *American Journal of Occupational Therapy* 32:565.

Hobson, D. A., and O. M. Nwaobi. 1985. The relationship between posture and ischial pressure for the high risk population. In *Proceedings, RESNA eighth annual conference*, 338-340. Washington, DC: RESNA Press.

Hobson, D. A., and R. E. Tooms. 1981. The foam-in-place seating system; Results of toxicity studies. In *Proceedings, RESNA fourth annual conference*, 45-48. Washington, DC: RESNA Press.

Kosiak, M. 1959. Etiology and pathology of ischemic ulcers. *Archives of Physical Medicine and Rehabilitation* 40:62.

Kosiak, M. 1976. A mechanical resting surface: Its effect on pressure distribution. *Archives of Physical Medicine and Rehabilitation* 57:481.

Krouskop, T. A., A. L. Muilenberg, D. R. Doughtery, and D. J. Winningham. 1987. Computer-aided design of a prosthetic socket for an above-knee amputee. *Journal of Rehabilitation Research and Development* 24:31.

Krouskop, T. A., P. C. Noble, S. L. Garber, and W. A. Spencer. 1983. The effectiveness of preventiveness management in reducing the recurrence of pressure sores. *Journal of Rehabilitation Research and Development* 20:174.

Noble, P. C., B. Goode, T. A. Krouskop, and B. Crisp. 1984. The influence of environmental aging upon the loadbearing properties of polyurethane foams. *Journal of Rehabilitation Research and Development* 21:31.

Perkash, I., H. O'Neill, D. Politi-Meeks, and C. L. Beets. 1984. Development and evaluation of a universal contoured cushion. *Paraplegia* 22:358.

Rodgers, J. E. 1974. Program for prevention of tissue breakdown. In *Report of progress of the rehabilitation engineering conference*, 50. Washington, DC: RESNA Press.

Shaw, C. G. 1988. *Improved seating for the elderly—Project 1: Needs assessment. Final report.* Memphis, TN: University of Tennessee.

Trefler, E., and J. Marcrum. 1987. Trends in powered mobility for school aged physically handicapped children. In *Proceedings, RESNA tenth annual conference*, 510-511. Washington, DC: RESNA Press.

Zackarkow, D. 1984. *Wheelchair posture and pressure sores.* Springfield, IL: Charles C. Thomas.

APPENDIX C

....

Problem-Solving Considerations

Appendix C
Problem-Solving Considerations

Problem	Possible Causes			Evaluation Review	Possible Solutions
	Neuromotor	Orthopedic	Functional/ Environmental		

I. Pelvis
 	
a. Posterior Tilt (sacral sitting— no lumbar curve)
	• central hypotonia
	• TLRP — > flexion
	• extensor thrust
		• tight hamstrings combined with:
		  —seat too long
		  —anterior wedge too high
		  —footrests too low
		• limited hip flexion
			• not seated far enough back in seat due to improper placement
			• seat belt too high (above ASIS)
				• determine appropriate orientation in space
				• review degree of hamstring tightness
					• Add knee block to maintain a neutral pelvic alignment if posture is not fixed
					• Tilt system back to decrease gravity's effect on the spine
					• Use lumbar/sacral pad
					• Alter position of head relative to position in space
					• Shorten seat depth, allowing knees to come under, if necessary; custom footrests to allow knees to flex
					• Decrease amount of wedging
					• Reposition pelvis, reinforce instructions to caregivers
					• Reposition lap belt

b. Lateral Tilt	• asymmetry of muscle tone	• scoliosis • subluxation/ dislocation of hip	• sling seat of wheelchair • seat too narrow	• evaluate flexibility of pelvis for possible realignment • review seating surface • review abnormal pathology • medical review for development of scoliosis/dislocated hip	• Solid seat with lateral pelvic blocks for midline orientation • Build up under buttock—low side if deformity is flexible, high side if deformity is fixed
c. Pelvic Rotation	• ATNR with rotation • asymmetry of muscle tone	• scoliosis with rota- tional component • thigh length discrepancy • subluxation/ dislocation of hip	• seat of chair fit for apparently longer thigh	• check to see if scoliosis is fixed or flexible • assess muscle tone and pathological reflexes	• Midline positioning of head to reduce the effects of ATNR • Midline, firm pelvic positioning • If fixed deformity, allow pelvis and lower extremities to rotate and to achieve forward position of head and trunk • With thigh length discrepancy, accommodate leg lengths individually

II. Hips					
a. Extension/ Adduction	• TLRS • positive supporting extensor thrust	• dislocation of hip(s)	• seat too short, causing inadequate pelvic/thigh support • hammocking of seat • insufficient hip flexion to overcome extensor tone	• check whether hip flexion results in adequate relaxation of adductors (may not be possible to gain correction with hip dislocation) • review position of body in space	• Seat depth 1½" shorter than "back of buttock to knee crease" measurement • Anterior wedge (usually 10 to 15 degrees with firm base) (hip flexion can facilitate abduction/external rotation pattern) Increase wedge depth only if no other way to control. With deeper wedges, watch length of sitting period in relation to circulation (compression on blood flow at hip/knee) • Remove footrest temporarily if necessary • Pommel—distal ⅓ of medial thigh • Ensure that head is in neutral orientation if TLRS is strong
b. Flexion/ Abduction	• primitive tonal patterns • hypotonic/athetoid • spastic flexion pattern • flexion/adduction internal rotation	• surgical adductor release	—	• review position of head in space	• Lateral thigh blocks maintain neutral with adequate stable base for sitting (30 to 40 degrees abduction) • Change functional work to eye level as much as possible
c. Internal/External Rotation	• abnormal tone • crossed extension reflex	• surgical abductor release	• may be stimulated by poor positioning of pelvis in seat • sling seat • improper pommel position combined with poor foot position	• if abduction/ adduction problems are corrected adequately, this should provide control needed	• Internal rotation—lateral extensions can be placed on footrest • Soft leg ties can sometimes be used • Neutral foot positioning often must block both laterally and medially to alleviate internal rotation posturing

Possible Causes

Problem	Neuromotor	Orthopedic	Functional/ Environmental	Evaluation Review	Possible Solutions
III. Spine a. Scoliosis	• hypotonia in trunk (muscles are not strong enough to override gravitational forces • asymmetrical muscle tone • ATNR • hypertonia or hypotonia	• fixed spinal deformity • pelvic obliquity/ asymmetry • see Pelvis section of this chart • tilt system (maintaining hip angle)	• functional demands	• evaluate for flexibility of curve • attempt correction and determine if forces required are realistic • check position of head to ATNR • medical review	• Powered or manual tilt system (maintaining hip angle) to decrease the effect of gravity on the trunk • Provide intimate trunk support using three-point pressure with some degree of recline if necessary • Firm midline positioning of pelvis and head • If having structural effect, change orientation or method of functional activity • See Pelvis section
b. Kyphosis	• posterior pelvic tilt • hypotonia in trunk • effect of STNR or TLRP • poor or no muscle resistance against gravity	• fixed spinal deformity	• seat depth too long • sling back • blindness	• determine flexibility of curve • determine effects of body-in-space changes • medical review	• Try a variety of anterior trunk supports • Lumbar/sacral supports • Accommodate back of system to support kyphosis if fixed • Sacral pads to alleviate posterior pelvic tilt • Tilt if fixed kyphosis
IV. Shoulder Girdle a. Retraction/ Adduction External Rotation	• TLRS • extensor thrust/ATNR • trunk hypotonia (instability of upper trunk causing "fixing" of shoulder girdle for stability)	— —	• instability of upper trunk, causing individual to attempt to "fix" proximally to gain stability • tray too high • system tilted too far	• review position of head relative to ATNR and TLS	• Decrease extensor tone • Alter position of head in space • Provide anterior chest support, tray positioned to weight bear with upper extremities for stabilization • Add protraction wings onto tray or back portion of seating system to assist in bringing arms to midline • May need pressure over shoulders to promote relaxation • Lower tray until shoulders are in a more neutral position

b. Protraction/ Adduction Internal Rotation	• TLRP	• kyphosis	• anterior shoulder restrains stimulating protraction	• as above • review best position for anterior restraints • check effects of increasing lumbar extension	• Alter position of head • Provide anterior trunk support • Raise tray height to assist with upper trunk extension • Provide lumbar/sacral support
V. Head and Neck a. Hyperextension	• extensor hypertonicity • poor flexor control • poor head control	—	• poor spinal alignment (that is, unaccommodated kyphosis) • poor headrest position	• review spinal alignment • check TLRP and STNR	• Stabilize trunk • Tilt in space if head/trunk control is poor to decrease the effects of gravity • Position head positioner below occipital region • Increase hip flexion and alleviate extensor tone • Provide lower work surface
b. Forward Flexion	• hypotonia (severe) • primitive flexor tone	• kyphosis	• headrest too far forward • back support too short • seating system too upright • work too low • severe/profound retardation with sensory deficits (cortical blindness)	• review spinal alignment • check TLS and STNR • tilt system in space	• Alter position in space (tilt back) • Alter headrest • Provide higher back • Provide higher or easel work surface • Provide anterior head support or chin support
c. Rotation	• ATNR • rooting reflex initiated by stimulation to cheek by neck collar	—	• auditory/ visual/ perceptual field deficits • position in relation to environmental stimulation (for example, stimulus all the way to the right of the client)	—	• Inhibit ATNR by midline head positioning • Larger, more supportive headrest • Avoid cheek area by selection of other type of head support • Reposition in environment

Possible Causes

Problem	Neuromotor	Orthopedic	Functional/Environmental	Evaluation Review	Possible Solutions
d. Lateral Flexion	• hydrocephalus (sign of increased intercranial pressure) • hypotonia	— —	• visual perceptual deficits	• observe behavior while repositioning head	• Get medical review • Midline positioning
VI. Lower Extremities **Knees** a. Flexion b. Extension	• tight hamstrings • part of total extension	• fixed deformities (contractures)	• inappropriate footrest • seat too short	• review effects of decreasing hip flexion angle	• Lengthen seat • Reduce hip flexion angle • Bevel front edge of seat to accommodate tight hamstrings
Feet a. Plantarflexion (with inversion)	• extensor patterns dominant • positive supporting reflex	• heelcord shortening • footrest too low	— —	• check whether sustained, or inhibited if maintained in flexion	• Add footstraps at 45 degrees • Raise footrests • Wedge footrests • Remove footrests temporarily • Wedge seat to decrease overall extensor tone • Accommodate/support
b. Dorsiflexion (with eversion)	• component of total flexor pattern	• hypersensitive plantar surface	• feet poorly supported	— —	• Accommodate and protect

Look to these products for current and comprehensive information . . .

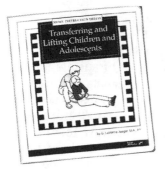

TRANSFERRING AND LIFTING CHILDREN AND ADOLESCENTS
Home Instruction Sheets
by D. LaVonne Jaeger, M.A., PT

Provide parents and caregivers of special needs children vital transportation guidance. You'll have 74 instruction sheets in forward-backward transfers, toileting, bathing, stairs, and mechanical lifting. Save time and money with this easy-to-use binder.

Catalog No. 4131-YTS $39

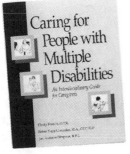

CARING FOR PEOPLE WITH MULTIPLE DISABILITIES
An Interdisciplinary Guide for Caregivers
by Cindy French, OTR, Robin T. Gonzalez, M.A., CCC-SLP, and Jan Tronson-Simpson, RPT

This reference guide gives caregivers a thorough understanding of therapeutic principles and their application. Explanations and illustrations of disabilities, daily-care techniques, and a glossary of common terms are included. Use reproducible forms and checklists for training and daily programming.

Catalog No. 4705-YTS $29.95

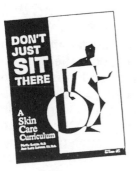

DON'T JUST SIT THERE
A Skin-Care Curriculum
by Martha Scotzin, Ph.D., and Joan Kurtz Sommer, M.A., RN

Teach your clients how to identify and treat pressure sores with this all-in-one skin-care program. You'll find applications to provide a sound base for starting a skin-care routine. Give your clients confidence to set individual goals with this video, manual, and client workbook.

Catalog No. 4742-YTS $125

ADULT POSITIONS, TRANSITIONS, AND TRANSFERS
Reproducible Instruction Cards for Caregivers
by Nancy Harris Ossman, OTR, and Marge Campbell, PT

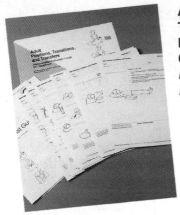

These reproducible cards show 28 positions, transitions, and transfers for your adult and geriatric clients. Each sturdy card gives step-by-step instructions and clear illustrations. You'll be able to remind caregivers how to help the patient develop good habits of movement and increase body awareness and self-control.

Catalog No. 4166-YTS $35

HOME CAREGIVER'S GUIDE
Articles for Adult Daily Living
by Jeffrey L. Crabtree, OTR, and Diane Crabtree, OTR

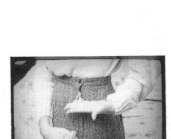

Address the concerns of caregivers of your geriatric clients with these reproducible articles. Provide home caregivers with easy-to-understand relevant care techniques for older adults with cognitive impairments or physical limitations. You'll have information on Taking Care of Personal Needs, and Living Well at Home.

Catalog No. 4222-YTS $49

ARTHRITIS AND EVERYDAY LIVING
by Cindy Collett Hodges, B.S., OTR

This one-of-a-kind video aids the professional, caregiver, and patient in the teaching, learning, and carryover of ADL techniques. Take your clients step-by-step through a daily living routine using this teaching aid. Clients learn energy conservation strategies to use when performing everyday household activities.

Catalog No. 4725-YTS $69

Order Form

Therapy Skill Builders
3830 E. Bellevue / P.O. Box 42050-YTS
Tucson, Arizona   85733

Ship to:

INSTITUTION: _____

NAME: _____

OCCUPATION/DEPARTMENT: _____

ADDRESS: _____

CITY:_____ STATE:_____ ZIP: _____

☐ Please check here if this is a permanent address change.
  If so, what was your previous zip code? _____

Telephone No._____   ☐ work ☐ home

Payment Options:

☐ My check is enclosed.

☐ My purchase order is enclosed. P.O.# _____
                                        (Net 30 days)

☐ Charge to my credit card.
  ☐ VISA   ☐ MasterCard   ☐ Discover

Card No. [ ][ ][ ][ ][ ][ ][ ][ ][ ][ ][ ][ ][ ][ ][ ][ ]

Expiration Date: Month_____   Year_____

Signature _____

Qty.	Cat. #	Title	Per	Amount
		SUBTOTAL		

Please add 10% for postage and assured delivery. 8% for orders over $500.
Arizona residents add sales tax.
Canada: Add 22% to subtotal for shipping, handling, and G.S.T.

Payment in U.S. funds only | **TOTAL** |

MONEY-BACK GUARANTEE
You'll have up to 90 days of risk-free evaluation
of the products you ordered. If you're not completely
satisfied with any product, we'll pick it up within
the 90 days and refund the full purchase price!
No Questions Asked!

FOR PHONE ORDERS
Call (602) 323-7500. Please have your
credit card and/or institutional purchase
order information ready.
9 AM–6 PM Central Time
Voice or TDD
FAX (602) 325-0306

We occasionally backorder items temporarily out of stock. If you do not accept backorders,
please tell us on your purchase order or on this form.